Studying a Study

and Testing a Test

How to Read
the Medical Literature

Studying a Study

and Testing a Test

HOW TO READ
THE MEDICAL LITERATURE
SECOND EDITION

Richard K. Riegelman, M.D., Ph.D.

Professor of Health Care Sciences and Medicine, Director, Master of Public Health Program, The George Washington University, School of Medicine and Health Sciences; Attending Physician, Department of Medicine, The George Washington University Hospital, Washington, D.C.

Robert P. Hirsch, Ph.D.

Associate Professor and Associate Chairman, Department of Health Care Sciences, The George Washington University, School of Medicine and Health Sciences, Washington, D.C.

Little, Brown and Company
Boston   Toronto   London

Library of Congress Catalog Card No. 89-84395

ISBN 0-316-74524-3

Printed in the United States of America

RRD VA

Contents

Preface

Faced with an onslaught of medical research what is the practicing clinician to do? How can we accurately and efficiently evaluate this information and incorporate it into clinical practice? The goal of *Studying a Study and Testing a Test: How to Read the Medical Literature*, Second Edition, is to teach a practical step-by-step approach to thoughtful, critical, and ultimately more efficient reading of the medical literature.

This second edition builds on the approaches used in the first edition. New material on controlled clinical trials examines what needs to be done and demonstrates what can go wrong in each step of the process. Flaw-catching exercises written for the second edition are included throughout the text. A reorganized and expanded flowchart of statistics summarizes the new chapters in Part 4, *Selecting a Statistic*. This second edition contains extensive footnotes designed for the statistically oriented reader or for formal classroom use. The basic text, however, remains oriented to clinicians who wish to read the literature on their own or as part of a journal club.

Statistical concepts are presented here, and their implications and assumptions are defined, but there is no undue emphasis on carrying out statistical manipulations. Instead, the emphasis is placed on clarifying the question that is being asked by a study, on determining whether a correct statistical test is being used, and on understanding the meaning of the results.

Experienced clinicians can pick up a two volume chart and systematically summarize the pertinent issues, yet they often have difficulty formally presenting a four page research paper. To deal with this need the reader of *Studying a Study and Testing a Test* is given uniform frameworks on which to build a critique of any research article. A checklist of questions for the reader to ask when evaluating a study also helps to develop a systematic approach that will speed up the process of analyzing articles.

Any useful approach to reading the medical literature must build on, and be compatible with, clinical training. In the differential diagnosis approach to clinical problems, an organized, structured framework helps clinicians to think through problems rapidly. Much as in learning to perform a physical examination, the reader's attention is directed initially to the individual components of the process. Capsule summaries of hypothetical journal articles that each focus on a particular type of error, illustrate and crystallize the essential concepts. The time spent in learning the basic principles results in the ability to comprehend more quickly the meaning and the limitations of any study one encounters.

The case study method used here is parallel to ward training or clinical/pathological conferences. It provides the active "hands on" training needed to internalize the concepts and gain proficiency in using them. At the end of the first three parts there are flaw-catching exercises—simulated articles fraught with a variety of errors that provide practice in applying the uniform framework. A sample critique of each flaw-catching exercise allows readers to evaluate the progress they are making in analyzing the material. A flowchart at the end of Part 4 summarizes the various statistical methods and guides the reader through the steps involved in statistical thinking. As in clinical training, the goal is an organized analysis of the data that will provide a basis for decision making.

The overall objective is to learn the kinds of questions that studies and statistics can answer as well as the kinds of questions we must answer for ourselves. It is important to recognize that studies that are less than ideal do not necessarily invalidate research or relieve clinicians of the responsibility to draw clinical conclusions. Clinicians who can critically read the medical literature and understand and accept the uncertainty that exists are better able to draw meaningful conclusions and integrate the results of medical research into clinical practice. Reading medical literature can be more than a responsibility. We hope we have taken some of the pain out of the process.

R.K.R.
R.P.H.

Acknowledgments

We are indebted to many persons who directly or indirectly contributed to this book. First and foremost, we would like to acknowledge the many medical and public health students who patiently tolerated our experimentation with methods of teaching epidemiology and medical statistics. Especially, we thank Sally Santen and Bob McNellis, students at The George Washington University, who read our manuscripts and provided many helpful suggestions. Also, we acknowledge the capable assistance of Yolanda Semonich who typed the manuscript and kept us on schedule, and Maureen Flaherty whose ability to organize long-term projects was invaluable. Finally, we express our deep appreciation to our families who endured long hours and working "vacations" necessary to complete this book.

Studying a Study

and Testing a Test

How to Read
the Medical Literature

PART 1

Studying a Study

CHAPTER 1

Introduction and Sample Test

The traditional course in reading the medical literature consists of "Here's the *New England Journal of Medicine*. Read it!" This approach is analogous to learning to swim by the total immersion method. Some persons can learn to swim this way, of course, but a few drown, and many learn to fear the water. Reading only the abstracts of medical articles is much like fearing the water.

In contrast to the method of total immersion, a step-by-step, active-participation approach to the review of the medical literature will be presented here. With these analytic techniques, the clinician should be able to read a journal article critically and efficiently. Considerable emphasis will be placed on the errors that can occur in the various kinds of studies, but try to remember that not every flaw is fatal.

Before developing and illustrating the elements of critical analysis, however, let us begin with a flaw-catching exercise, a simulated journal article, and see how well you can do. Read the following study and then try to answer the accompanying questions.

A STUDY OF MEDICAL SCREENING IN A MILITARY POPULATION

During their first year in the military service, 10,000 eighteen-year-old privates were offered the opportunity to participate in a yearly health maintenance examination that included history, physical examination, and multiple laboratory tests. The first year 5,000 participated and 5,000 failed to participate. The 5,000 participants were selected as a study group, and the 5,000 nonparticipants were selected as a control group. The first-year participants were then offered yearly health maintenance examinations during each year of their military service.

On discharge from the military, each of the 5,000 study group members and each of the 5,000 control group members were given an extensive history, physical examination, and laboratory evaluation to determine whether the yearly health maintenance visits had made any difference in health and life-style of the participants.

The investigators obtained the following information:

1. On the basis of their reported consumption, participants had half the rate of alcoholism as nonparticipants.
2. Participants had twice as many diagnoses made on them during military service as nonparticipants.
3. Participants had advanced an average of twice as many ranks as nonparticipants.
4. No statistically significant differences occurred between the groups in the rate of myocardial infarction (MI).
5. No differences were found between the groups in the rate of development of testicular cancer or Hodgkin's disease, the two most common cancers in young men.

The authors then drew the following conclusions:

1. Yearly screening can reduce the rate of alcoholism in the entire military by one-half.
2. Since participants had twice the number of diagnoses made on them, their diseases were being diagnosed at an earlier stage in the disease process, at a point where therapy is more beneficial.
3. Since participants had twice the military advancement of nonparticipants, the screening program must have contributed to the quality of their work.
4. Since no differences occurred between the groups in the rate of MI, screening and intervention for coronary risk factors should not be included in a future health maintenance screening program.
5. Since testicular cancer and Hodgkin's disease occurred with equal frequency in both groups, future health maintenance examinations should not include efforts to diagnose these conditions.

Now see if you can answer the following questions, which form the uniform framework for reviewing medical studies.

1. Was the study properly designed to answer the study questions?
2. Was the method of assignment of patients to the study and control groups proper?

3. Was the assessment of the results in the study group and in the control group adequately performed?
4. Did the analysis properly compare the outcome in the study and the control groups?
5. Was a valid interpretation drawn from the comparisons made between the study and control groups?
6. Were the extrapolations to individuals not involved in the study properly performed?

How did you do? If you feel you can answer these questions already, turn to the critique on page 88 and compare your answers. When you are ready, let us proceed!

CHAPTER 2

Uniform Frameworks

UNIFORM FRAMEWORK

Three basic types of clinical research studies are frequently found in the medical literature: case-control or retrospective studies, cohort studies or prospective studies, and randomized clinical trials or controlled clinical trials. A uniform framework can be used to evaluate all three types of studies. It will constitute the foundation for the entire process of studying a study. Figure 2-1 outlines the application of the uniform framework to a research study.

The uniform framework contains the following basic components:

ASSIGNMENT   Selection of individuals for study and control groups

ASSESSMENT   Determination of the results of the investigation in the study and the control groups

ANALYSIS   Comparison of the results of the study and the control groups

INTERPRETATION   Drawing conclusions about the meaning of and differences found between the study and the control groups for those in the study

EXTRAPOLATION   Drawing conclusions about the meaning of the study for individuals or situations not included in the study

In order to illustrate the application of the uniform framework to case-control (retrospective), cohort (prospective), and randomized clinical trial (controlled clinical trial) studies, let us outline the essential features of each type of study and then see how we could apply each type of study to the specific problem of the relationship between unopposed estrogen use (estrogen without progesterone) and endometrial cancer.

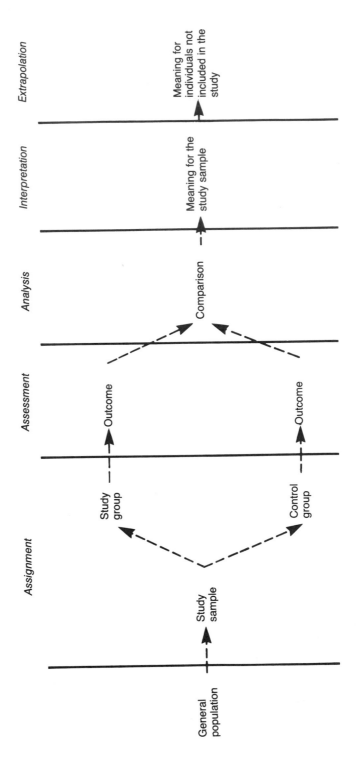

FIGURE 2-1 *Uniform framework for studying a study.*

Case-Control Study (Retrospective Study)

The unique feature of *case-control studies,* or *retrospective studies,* is that they begin after individuals already have developed or failed to develop the disease being investigated. They go back in time to determine the characteristics of individuals prior to the onset of disease. In case-control studies "cases" are the individuals who have developed the disease already, and the controls are the individuals who have not developed the disease. In order to use a retrospective study to examine the relationship between unopposed estrogen use and endometrial cancer, an investigator would proceed as follows:

ASSIGNMENT   Select a study group of women who currently have endometrial cancer (cases) and a group of otherwise similar women who do not have endometrial cancer (controls). Since the development of the disease has occurred without the investigator's intervention, this process is called *observed assignment.*

ASSESSMENT   Determine whether each woman in the study group and in the control group previously took unopposed estrogens and, if so, assess how much she used.

ANALYSIS   Calculate the odds that the group of women with endometrial cancer had used unopposed estrogens versus the odds that the group of women without endometrial cancer had used unopposed estrogens.

INTERPRETATION   Draw conclusions about the meaning of unopposed estrogen use for women included in the study.

EXTRAPOLATION   Draw conclusions about the meaning of estrogen use for categories of women not included in the study such as other women on the same or different dosages or combined use of estrogen and progesterone. Figure 2-2 illustrates the application of the uniform framework to this study.

Cohort Study (Prospective Study)

Cohort studies, or *prospective studies,* differ from case-control studies in that they begin before individuals have developed the disease that is being investigated and follow them forward in time to determine who subsequently will develop the disease. A *cohort* is a group of individuals who share a common experience. Cohort or prospective studies follow a cohort that possesses the characteristics under study as well as a cohort that does not possess that particular characteristic. In order to use a cohort study to examine the relationship between unopposed estrogen use and endometrial cancer, an investigator would proceed as follows:

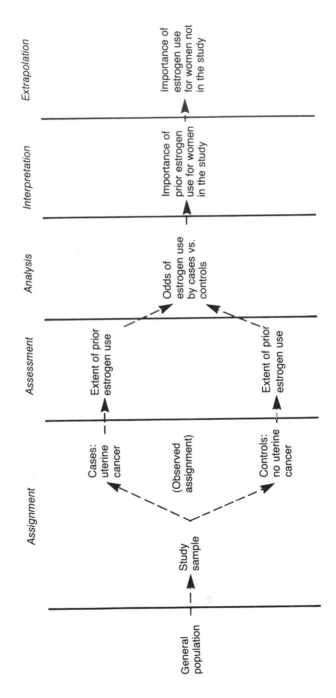

FIGURE 2-2 *Application of the uniform framework to a case-control or retrospective study.*

ASSIGNMENT   Select a study group of women who are using unopposed estrogens and an otherwise similar control group of women who are not and have not used unopposed estrogens. Since the use of unopposed estrogens is observed to occur without the investigator's intervention, this process is also called observed assignment.

ASSESSMENT   Follow the study group and the control groups of women to determine who subsequently develops endometrial cancer.

ANALYSIS   Calculate the probability of developing endometrial cancer for women using unopposed estrogens versus women not using estrogens.

INTERPRETATION   Draw conclusions about the meaning of unopposed estrogen use for women included in the study.

EXTRAPOLATION   Draw conclusions about the use of unopposed estrogens for women not included in the study such as women on the same or different dosages or combined use of estrogen and progesterone. Figure 2-3 illustrates the application of the uniform framework to a cohort or prospective study.

Randomized Clinical Trial (Controlled Clinical Trial)

Randomized clinical trials are also called *controlled clinical trials*. As in cohort studies, individuals are followed forward in time to determine if they develop a particular disease or condition under investigation. The unique feature of experimental studies, however, is the method for assigning individuals to study and control groups. Ideally, individuals are randomized and assigned blindly either to a study group or to a control group. *Randomization* means that any one individual has a known probability of being assigned to the study or the control group. *Double-blind assignment,* the preferred form of blinding, means that neither the participants nor the investigators know whether a particular participant has been assigned to a study or to a control group. To use a randomized clinical trial to examine the relationship between unopposed estrogens and endometrial cancer, an investigator would proceed as follows:

ASSIGNMENT   Using randomization, women are blindly assigned to a study group that will use unopposed estrogen or to a nonestrogen-taking control group.

ASSESSMENT   Follow these women forward in time to determine who subsequently develops uterine cancer.

ANALYSIS   Calculate the probability of women using estrogen developing endometrial cancer versus women not using estrogen.

INTERPRETATION   Draw conclusions about the meaning of the unopposed estrogen use for women included in the study.

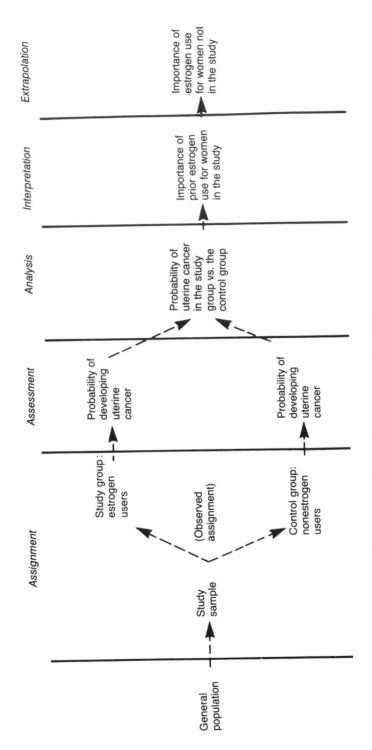

FIGURE 2-3 *Application of the uniform framework to a cohort or prospective study.*

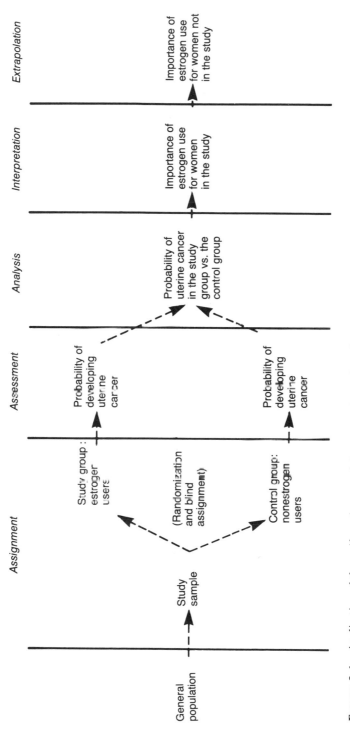

FIGURE 2-4 Application of the uniform framework to an experimental study.

EXTRAPOLATION   Draw conclusions about the meaning of unopposed estrogen use for women not included in the study such as women on different dosages or combined use of estrogen and progesterone. Figure 2-4 illustrates the application of the uniform framework to the randomized clinical trial or controlled clinical trial.

This brief presentation of the three basic study types used in clinical studies is designed to show how each type of study can be analyzed by using the uniform framework. In Chapter 8, the strength and weakness of each study type will be discussed. Before proceeding further with overall study design, however, let us discuss the requirements for proper implementation of each component in the uniform framework and illustrate the common errors that can occur.

CHAPTER 3

Assignment

OBSERVATIONAL STUDIES

In the next six chapters we apply our uniform framework to case-control and cohort studies. Together these types of studies are known as *observational studies*. In an observational study no intervention is attempted, and no attempt is made to alter the course of a disease. The investigators observe the course of the disease among groups with and without the characteristics being studied.

Investigations are generally conducted using a sample or subgroup of individuals chosen from a larger population. The individuals chosen may or may not be randomly selected from a larger population using a chance process. Thus, the study and control groups are not necessarily representative of all those in a larger population. The characteristics of the individuals eligible for the study and control groups, however, are defined by the investigator with an aim to create study and control groups that are as identical as possible except for the characteristic(s) under study. The presence of selection bias is one reason that this goal may not be fulfilled.

Few terms used in medicine are less clearly understood or more loosely used than the word *bias*. *Webster's New World Dictionary* defines *bias* as "prejudice, a judgment or opinion formed before the facts are known."* According to the best tradition of scientific research, a study should be free of prejudice. Yet, even with the best of scientific intentions, investigators can unintentionally introduce factors into the

---

* *Webster's New World Dictionary of the American Language. (College Edition).* Cleveland: World Publishing Company, 1966. p. 1150.

investigation that predetermine the outcome of the study. The presence of these factors may create a selection bias. The elements of selection bias are illustrated in the following hypothetical study:*

A case-control study of the causes of premenopausal breast cancer compared the past use of birth control pills among 500 females with breast cancer to the past use of the pill among 500 age-matched women admitted for hypertension or diabetes. Investigators found that 40% of the women with breast cancer had used birth control pills during the preceding 5 years while only 5% of those with diabetes or hypertension in the control group had used the pill. The authors concluded that a strong association existed between the use of birth control pills and the development of premenopausal breast cancer.

In order to determine whether a selection bias may have existed in the assignment of patients to the control group, one must first ask whether patients in the control group were similar to the total population of women without breast cancer. The answer is no, since these women were unique in being admitted to the hospital for diabetes or hypertension. One must then ask whether their uniqueness was likely to have affected their use of the characteristic under study, that is, birth control pills. The answer is yes. Since birth control pills are widely known to increase blood pressure and blood sugar, physicians are not likely to prescribe birth control pills to women with hypertension and diabetes. Thus the uniqueness of the health of these women contributed to a lower-than-expected use of birth control pills. This study, therefore, created the potential for a selection bias in the assignment of patients.

Thus selection bias can occur whenever the study and control groups differ from each other by a factor that is likely to affect the outcome measure being studied. In other words selection bias occurs when the groups differ in a way that makes a difference in the outcome.

Selection bias can occur in a cohort study as illustrated in the following example:

The effect of cigarette smoking on the development of myocardial infarctions was studied by selecting 10,000 cigarette smokers and 10,000 noncigarette-smoking pipe smokers. Both groups were followed for 10 years. The investigators found that the cigarette smokers had a rate of new myocardial infarction of 4 per 100 over 10 years while the noncigarette-smoking pipe smokers had a rate of new myocardial infarction of 7 per 100 over 10 years. The results were statistically significant. The investigators concluded that cigarette smokers have

---

* In reviewing this hypothetical case as well as the others in the book, the reader should assume that all omitted portions of the study were properly performed.

a lower risk of myocardial infarctions than noncigarette-smoking pipe smokers.

Despite the statistical significance of this difference, the conclusion is in conflict with the results of many other studies. Let us see if selection bias could have contributed to the results.

In analyzing this study, one must recognize two generally accepted facts: Men make up the vast majority of pipe smokers, and men have a much higher rate of myocardial infarction than women.

With these facts in mind, the first question to ask is whether the study and control groups differ. The answer is yes, since men constitute the vast majority of pipe smokers whereas more women smoke cigarettes than pipes. To establish the potential for a selection bias we must also ask would this difference affect the outcome being measured. Again the answer is yes. Men have a higher risk of myocardial infarction. Thus both elements of selection bias are present. The groups differ in a way that makes a difference.

Even when selection bias is unlikely, chance alone may produce study and control groups that differ according to risk factors for development of disease or prognostic factors that affect the outcome of the disease. When these differences in risk factors affect outcome, they are known as *confounding variables*. Thus, a selection bias is a special case of a confounding variable, which results from bias in the way the study or the control group subjects are selected. Remember, even in the absence of selection bias, differences in confounding variables can result by chance alone. It is important to compare the study and the control group subjects to determine if they differ in ways that are likely to affect outcome. In Chapters 5 and 29 we discuss methods that may be used to prevent or deal with confounding variables, but first let us take a look at the type of problems that can occur in assessment of outcome.

CHAPTER 4

Assessment of Outcome

To assess the outcome of an investigation, researchers must define the *outcome* or *end point* that they intend to measure. The term *outcome* can be somewhat confusing because it has different meanings for the different types of studies. Let us review what *outcome* means in case-control and cohort studies and then define the criteria for a valid measure of outcome. Cohort studies begin with a study group that possesses the characteristic under study and a control group that is free of this characteristic. Individuals in the study and control groups are followed forward in time to determine whether they will develop a particular condition. The occurrence of the condition that is being assessed is known as the outcome or end point.

The investigator must employ a valid measure of the occurrence of the condition. For instance, in the unopposed estrogen and endome trial cancer examples, the development of endometrial cancer is the outcome being assessed by the investigators.

Case-control studies begin with persons who have already developed a certain condition (cases) and persons who have not developed the condition (controls). The investigators review the past history of the individuals in both the case and the control groups to determine whether these individuals had exposure to, or possession of, a prior characteristic. In a case-control study, this prior characteristic is the outcome of the study. A valid measure of the outcome or prior characteristic must be employed by investigators. In the case of the unopposed estrogens and endometrial cancer example, the use of unopposed estrogens is the characteristic being assessed.

What constitutes a proper measure of outcome? Each of the following criteria must be satisfied:

1. The investigator must use a measure that is appropriate to the question being addressed.
2. The measure of outcome must be accurate. It must approximate true measurement of the phenomenon.
3. The measure of outcome must be complete.
4. The study's measure of the outcome must not be influenced by the process of observation.

APPROPRIATE MEASURE OF OUTCOME

To understand the importance of the appropriateness of a measure of outcome, let us first consider an example of how the use of an inappropriate measure of outcome can invalidate a study's conclusions.

An investigator attempted to study whether users of brand A or brand B spermicide had a lower probability of developing tubal infections due to *Chlamydia*. The investigator identified 100 women using each brand of spermicide, followed these women, and did cervical cultures for *Chlamydia*, on a yearly basis for 5 years. The investigator found that women using brand A spermicide had 1½ times as many positive cultures for *Chlamydia*. The investigator concluded that brand B spermicide is associated with a lower rate of tubal infections.

Chlamydia cultures from the cervix do little to establish the presence or absence of tubal infection. The study may help to establish a higher frequency of *Chlamydia* infection. However, if the intent is to study the relative frequency of tubal infection, the investigator has not chosen an appropriate outcome measurement or endpoint.

ACCURATE MEASURE OF OUTCOME

Next we will look at how an outcome assessment may be affected by inaccurate measurements. Information for measuring outcome may come from three sources:

1. Readings from testing instruments
2. Measurements by the study investigator
3. Reports or records from individuals

The information obtained may be inaccurate because it produces data that are always off-target in the same direction, due to bias in the way the data are collected. Alternatively, data may be inaccurate because of chance variation in either direction.

Information from study individuals is subject to recall and reporting bias. *Recall bias* implies defects in memory, especially defects in which one group is more likely to recall events than other groups. *Reporting bias* occurs in a case-control study when one group of study subjects is more accurate than the other in reporting what they remember. Consider the following example of how recall bias can occur:

In a case-control study of the cause of spina bifida, 100 mothers of infants born with the disease and 100 mothers of infants born without the disease are studied. Of the mothers of spina bifida infants, 50% reported having had a sore throat during pregnancy versus 5% of the mothers whose infants did not develop spina bifida. The investigators concluded that they had shown an association between sore throats during pregnancy and spina bifida.

Before accepting the conclusions of the study, one must ask whether recall bias could explain its findings. One can argue that mothers who experienced the trauma of having an infant with spina bifida are likely to search their memory more intensively and to remember events not usually recalled by other women. Thus recall bias is more likely to occur when the subsequent events are traumatic, thereby causing subjectively remembered and frequently occurring events to be recalled, which under normal circumstances would be forgotten. Therefore, the result of this case-control study may be attributable, at least in part, to recall bias. The potential for recall bias casts doubts on the alleged association between sore throats and the occurrence of spina bifida.

Reporting bias as well as recall bias may operate to impair the accuracy of the outcome assessment as illustrated in the following example:

A study of the relationship between gonorrhea and multiple sexual partners was conducted. One hundred women who were newly diagnosed as having gonorrhea were compared with 100 women in the same clinic who were found to be free of gonorrhea. The women who were diagnosed as having gonorrhea were informed that the serious consequences of the disease could be prevented only by locating and treating their sexual partners. Both groups of women were asked about the number of sexual partners they had during the preceding two months. The group of women with gonorrhea reported an average of twice as many sexual partners as the group of women without gonorrhea. The investigators concluded that women with gonorrhea have twice as many sexual partners as women without gonorrhea.

It can be argued that the women with gonorrhea in this study felt a greater obligation, hence less hesitation, to report their sexual partners than did the women without the disease. Reporting bias is more likely to occur when the information sought is personal or sensitive.

In addition, one group is under more pressure than another to report previous events accurately. Thus, it is possible that women with gonorrhea may simply have been more thorough in reporting their sexual partners rather than actually having more contacts. Reporting error in conjunction with recall error may impair the accuracy of assessment in case-control studies.

Instrument Error

Error in measurement may also occur as a result of inaccurate measurement by the testing instruments, as illustrated in the following example:

The gastrointestinal side effects of two nonsteroidal anti-inflammatory medications for arthritis were assessed by use of an upper gastrointestinal x ray. The investigator found no evidence that either drug was associated with gastritis.

The investigator did not recognize that an upper GI x ray is a very poor instrument for measuring gastritis. Even if a drug caused gastritis, upper GI x-ray examination would not be adequate to identify its presence. Thus any conclusion based on this measurement is likely to be inaccurate. When gross instrument error occurs, as in this example, the measurement of outcome also can be considered inappropriate.

Investigator Bias

Whenever the measurement of outcome depends on subjective interpretation of data, the possibility of investigator bias exists. It is possible, however, to recognize and correct for a fundamental principle of human psychology, namely, that persons, including investigators, see what they want to see or expect to see. This is accomplished by keeping the investigator, who makes the assessment of outcome, from knowing an individual's group assignment. Blind assessment can be used in case-control and cohort studies as well as randomized clinical trials. Failure to use blind assessment can lead to the following type of bias:

In a study of the use of nonsteroidal anti-inflammatory drugs, the investigators, who were the patients' attending physicians, questioned all patients to determine whether one of the nonsteroidals was associated with more symptoms compatible with gastritis. After questioning all patients about their symptoms, they determined that there was no difference in the occurrence of gastritis. They reported that the two drugs produced the same occurrence of gastritis symptoms.

In this study the investigators making the assessment of outcome were aware of what the patients were receiving, thus they were not "blinded." In addition, they were assessing the patients' subjective symptoms such as nausea, stomach pain, or indigestion in deciding whether gastritis was present. This is the setting in which blinding is most critical. Even if the patients were unaware of which medication they were on, the investigators' assessment may be biased. If the assessment conformed with their own hypothesis, their results are especially open to question. This does not imply fraud, only the natural tendency of human beings to see what they expect or want to see. The investigators' conclusions may be true, but their less-than-perfect techniques make it difficult or impossible to accept their conclusion. Thus blinding in the process of assessment is important to eliminate bias.

COMPLETENESS OF ASSESSMENT

Whenever follow-up of patients is incomplete, the possibility exists that those not included in the final assessment had a different frequency of outcome from those included. The following example illustrates an error due to incomplete assessment:

A cohort study of human immunodeficiency virus (HIV)-positive patients compared the natural history of the disease among asymptomatic patients with a T4 count of 100 to 200 compared to a group of asymptomatic HIV-positive patients with a T4 count of 200 to 400. The investigators were able to follow-up 50% of those with the lower T4 counts and 60% of those with the high T4 counts. The investigators found no difference between the groups and concluded that the T4 count is not a risk factor for developing acquired immunodeficiency syndrome (AIDS).

It can be argued that in this study, a number of those who could not be followed-up were not available because they were dead. If this were the case, the results of the study might have been dramatically altered with complete follow-up. Incomplete follow-up can distort the conclusions of an investigation.

Incomplete follow-up does not necessarily mean that the patients are lost to follow-up as in the previous example. They may be followed to varying extents as the next example illustrates:

A cohort study of the side effects of birth control pills was conducted by comparing 1,000 young women on the pill with 1,000 young women on other forms of birth control. Data were collected from the records of their private physicians over a 1-year period. Pill users were scheduled for three follow-up visits during the year; other women were asked to return if they had problems. Among users of the pill, 75 women reported having headaches, 90 reported fatigue, and 60 reported depression. Among nonpill users, 25 patients reported having headaches, 30 reported fatigue, and 20 reported depression. The average pill user made three visits to her physician during the year versus one visit for the nonpill user. The investigator concluded that use of the pill is associated with increased frequency of headaches, fatigue, and depression.

The problem of unequal observation of the two groups may have invalidated the results. The fact that pill users made 3 times as many visits to the physician may account for the more frequent recordings of headaches, fatigue, and depression. With more frequent observation, frequently occurring subjective symptoms are more likely to be reported.

EFFECT OF OBSERVATION

Even if a study's end point meets the difficult criteria of appropriate, accurate, and complete assessment, one more area of concern exists. Investigators intend to measure events as they would have occurred had no one been watching. Unfortunately, the very process of conducting a study may involve the introduction of an observer into the events being measured. Thus, the reviewer must determine whether the process of observation altered the outcome. An example follows in which this may have occurred:

A cohort study was conducted of the relationship between obesity and menstrual regularity. One thousand obese women with menstrual irregularities who had joined a diet group were compared with 1,000 obese women with the same pattern of menstrual irregularities who were not enrolled in a diet group. The women were compared to evaluate the effects of weight loss on menstrual irregularities. Those in the diet group had exactly the same frequency of return to regular menstrual cycles as the nondiet group controls.

It is possible that the nondiet group patients lost weight just like the diet group patients since they were being observed as part of the study. Whenever it is possible for subjects to switch groups or alter their behavior, the effects of observation may affect an investigation. This is most likely to occur when the control group patients are aware of adverse consequences of their current behavior and are placed under direct or indirect pressure to change by the process of observation.

CHAPTER 5

Analysis

In this chapter we introduce three fundamental roles of analysis:

1. To remove the effects of confounding variables
2. To test hypotheses that allow the investigator to draw conclusions regarding differences between large populations based on samples of the populations
3. To measure the size of the differences between groups or the strengths of the relationship between variables found in the study

As we discussed in Chapter 3, confounding variables can result from either chance or bias. Chance is an inherent problem whenever we obtain samples of large populations and desire to draw conclusions about the large population. As opposed to bias, the effect of chance is unpredictable.* It may either favor or oppose the study hypothesis in a way that cannot be predicted beforehand.

Bias, on the other hand, implies a systematic effect on the data in one particular direction that predictably favors or opposes the study hypothesis. Bias results from the way the patients were assigned or assessed.

Bias and chance may each produce differences among confounding variables resulting in study and control groups that differ in ways that can affect the outcome of the study. Let us begin our discussion of analyses by examining the available techniques for dealing with confounding variables. The basic techniques for removing the effects of

---

* Some effects of chance are predictable (e.g., imprecise determination of disease status in a case-control study will cause the odds to be underestimated).

bias are matching or pairing of study and control samples at the beginning of the study or adjustment of the data as part of the analysis.

PRIOR MATCHING

One method for circumventing the problem of confounding variables is to match individuals who are similar with respect to a potential confounding variable. For instance, if age is related to the probability of getting into either group, and if age is also related to outcome, then the investigator may match for age. For every 65-year-old in the control group, investigators could choose one 65-year-old for the study group, and similarly with 30-year-olds, 40-year-olds, and so on. If properly performed, the result of matching guarantees that the distribution of ages in each group will be the same.

Matching is not limited to making the groups uniform for age. It may be used for any factor that is a risk or prognostic factor, that is, a factor related to the probability of experiencing the outcome under study. Matching is especially useful to diminish the likelihood of selection bias. For example, if one were studying the relationship between birth control pills and strokes, then blood pressure would be considered an important risk or prognostic factor. Since high blood pressure is a relative contraindication to the use of birth control pills, high blood pressure should lower the probability that a women is on birth control pills. In addition, since high blood pressure also is known to increase the probability of strokes, high blood pressure also would affect the probability of developing the outcome. Therefore, blood pressure is a confounding variable on which one might want to match the groups.

One disadvantage of matching groups is that the investigators cannot study the effects on the outcome of the factor on which they matched the groups.* For instance, if they match for age and blood pressure, they lose the ability to study the effect of age and blood pressure on the development of strokes. Furthermore, they lose the ability to study factors that are closely associated with the matched factor. The pitfall in attempting to study the matched factor or closely linked factors is illustrated in the following example:

One hundred adult-onset diabetics were compared with one hundred non-diabetic adults to study factors associated with adult-onset diabetes. The groups were matched to ensure a similar weight distribution in the two groups. The authors also found that the total calo-

---

* The variables being matched can still be studied in terms of their interaction with other characteristics.

ries consumed in each of the two groups was nearly identical and concluded that the number of calories consumed was not related to the possibility of developing adult-onset diabetes.

The authors of the study, having matched the patients by weight, then attempted to study the differences in calories consumed. Since there is a high level of correlation between weight and calories consumed, it is not surprising that the authors found no difference in consumption of calories between the two groups matched for weight. It is not possible to investigate the possibility that matching factors or factors closely associated with the matched factors are associated with the occurrence of the outcome.

The type of matching discussed in our diabetes example is called *group matched*. A second type of matching is also known as *pairing* (i.e., when one study and one control group are included in an investigation). Pairing involves identifying one individual in the study group who can be compared to one or more individuals in the control group. Pairing of individuals is a very effective method of eliminating bias.

Despite the advantages of pairing, it has a distinct disadvantage. It may often be a problem to identify a control group patient who possesses all the same known risk factors as the study subject used in the pair. At times this problem can be circumvented by using a patient as his or her own control. This may be done in what is called a *cross-over study* in which the same individuals are compared to themselves while on and off the medication. When properly performed, these types of studies allow one to use the same individuals in the study group and control group and pair their results, thus keeping many factors constant. Since the individual is his or her own control, pairing allows the use of powerful statistical significance tests that have an increased probability of demonstrating statistical significance for a particular size study group. These are usually called *matched* tests.

Cross-over studies must be used with great care, however, or they can produce misleading results as the following hypothetical study illustrates:

A study of the benefit of a new non-narcotic medication for postoperative pain relief was performed by giving 100 patients the medication on day 1 postoperative and a placebo on day 2. For each patient the degree of pain was measured on a well-established pain scale on day 1 and day 2. The investigators found no difference between levels of pain on and off the medication.

When evaluating a cross-over design, one must recognize the potential for an effect of time and a carry-over effect of treatment. Pain is expected to decrease with time after surgery so it is not fair to compare the degree of pain on day 1 to the degree of pain on day 2.

Furthermore one must be careful to assess whether there may be a carry-over effect in which the medication on day 1 continues to be active on day 2. Thus the absence of benefit in this cross-over trial should not imply that pain medication on day 1 after surgery is no more effective than placebo.

STATISTICAL SIGNIFICANCE TESTING

Most investigations are conducted on only a sample or subset of the larger group of individuals who could have been included in the study. Researchers therefore are frequently confronted with the question of whether they would achieve similar results if the larger population were used or whether chance selection has produced unusual results in their particular sample. Unfortunately, there is no direct method for answering this question. Instead, investigators are forced to test their study hypothesis using a circuitous method of proof by elimination. This method is known as *statistical significance testing*.

Statistical significance testing, in its most common form, quantitates from the study data the probability of obtaining the observed data or a more extreme result if no associations between factors actually exist in the larger population. Statistical significance testing assumes that individuals used in an investigation are representative or randomly selected from a larger population. This use of the term *random* is confusing because statistical significance testing is used in studies in which the individuals assigned to a study or a control group are not randomly selected. This apparent contradiction can be reconciled if one regards the larger population as made up of individuals with the same characteristics as those required for entry into the study. Thus statistical significance tests are really addressing questions about larger populations made up of individuals just like the ones used in the investigation.

Statistical Significance Testing Procedures

Statistical significance testing or hypothesis testing is based on the premise that the world consists of two types of relationships: Either two factors are associated, or they are not associated. These factors, also called characteristics or variables, are associated if they occur together more often than expected by chance alone. The role of statistical significance testing or hypothesis testing is to determine whether the results are so unusual, if an association does not actually exist, that we are willing to assume an association exists. However, in statistical significance testing, one assumes at the beginning that no association exists. Notice that the issue is whether or not an association exists. Statistical significance testing itself says nothing about the strength or importance of the potential association.

Statistical significance testing begins with a study hypothesis stating that an association of factors exists in the larger population. In performing statistical significance tests, it is assumed initially that the study hypothesis is false, and a null hypothesis is formulated stating that no difference or association exists in the larger population. Statistical methods then are used to calculate the probability of obtaining the observed results in the study sample or more extreme results if no association actually exists in the larger population.

When only a small probability exists that the observed results would occur if the null hypothesis were true, then investigators can reject the contention that the null hypothesis is true and reject the null hypothesis. In rejecting the null hypothesis, the investigators accept by elimination the existence of their only other alternative— the existence of an association or difference between the larger population(s). The specific steps in statistical significance testing proceed as follows:

1. State hypothesis: Before collecting the data, the investigators state a study hypothesis that a difference exists between the study group and the control group.

2. Formulate null hypothesis: The investigators then assume that no true difference exists between the study group and the control group This is known as the null hypothesis.

3. Decide statistical significance level: The investigators determine what level of probability will be considered small enough to reject the null hypothesis. In a majority of medical research studies, a 5% chance or less of occurrence is considered unlikely enough to allow the investigators to reject the null hypothesis. The 5% figure is traditional. However, as with any level, we are left with some possibility that chance alone has produced an unusual set of data. Thus a null hypothesis, which is in fact true, may be rejected in favor of the study hypothesis as much as 5% of the time.

4. Collect data: The data may be collected using study designs such as a case-control, cohort, or randomized clinical trial.

5. Apply statistical significance test: If differences between the sample groups exist, the investigators determine the probability that these

differences would occur if no true differences exist in the larger populations from which both the study and control group individuals have been selected. This probability is known as the P value. In other words, they calculate the probability that the observed data or more extreme data would occur if the null hypothesis of no difference were true. In order to do so, the investigators must choose from among a variety of statistical significance tests, each one of which is appropriate to a specific type of data. Therefore, investigators must be careful that they have chosen the proper test, as we discuss in Chapters 27 through 30.

To understand how a statistical significance test measures probability or P values, let us look at an example that uses numbers small enough to allow for easy calculation. Assume that an investigator wants to study the question *"Are there an equal number of males and females born in the United States?"* The investigator first hypothesizes that more males than females are born in the United States; he then formulates a null hypothesis that an equal number of males and females are born in the United States. Then he decides the statistical significance level, which is usually set at 5% or $P = 0.05$. Next, he samples four birth certificates and finds that there are four males and zero females in his sample of births. Let us now calculate the probability of obtaining four males and zero females if the null hypothesis of equal numbers of males and females is true:

Probability of one male	0.50	or 50%
Probability of two males in a row	0.25	or 25%
Probability of three males in a row	0.125	or 12.5%
Probability of four males in a row	0.0625	or 6.25%

Thus there is a 6.25% chance of obtaining four males in a row even if an equal number of males and females are born in the United States. Thus the "P value" equals .0625.* A simple form of statistical significance test such as this one can yield the probability of producing the observed data, assuming that the null hypothesis is true. Most statistical significance tests yield similar types of results. They all measure the probability of obtaining the observed data or more extreme data if no true differences between groups actually exist in the larger populations.

6. Reject or fail to reject the null hypothesis: Having determined the probability that the results could have occurred by chance if no true differences exist in the larger population, the investigators proceed

---

* We have calculated a one-tailed statistical significance test.

to reject or fail to reject the null hypothesis. If the probability of the results occurring by chance is less than or equal to 0.05, investigators can reject the null hypothesis, thereby indicating that the probability is small enough that chance alone is not likely to explain the differences. By elimination they accept the proposition that a true difference exists in the outcome between the larger population of study individuals and the larger population of control individuals from which the research individuals were selected.

What if the probability of occurrence by chance is greater than 0.05 as in the preceding example? The investigators then are unable to reject the null hypothesis. This does not mean that the null hypothesis that no true difference in the larger population is true or even likely. It merely indicates that the probability of obtaining the observed results, if the null hypothesis were true, is too great to reject the null hypothesis in favor of the study hypothesis. The burden of proof, therefore, is on the investigators to show that the null hypothesis is quite unlikely before rejecting it in favor of the study hypothesis. The following example shows how the significance testing procedure operates in practice:

An investigator wanted to test the hypothesis that mouth cancer is associated with pipe smoking. She formulated a null hypothesis stating that pipe smoking is not associated with mouth cancer in the general population. She then decided that if she obtained data that would occur only 5% or less of the time if the null hypothesis were true, she would reject the null hypothesis. She next collected data from a sample of the general population of pipe smokers and non-smokers. Using the proper statistical significance test, she found that if no association existed between pipe smoking and mouth cancer in the general population, then data as extreme or more extreme than her data would be observed by chance only 3% of the time. She now concluded that since her data were quite unlikely to occur if there were no association between pipe smoking and mouth cancer, she would reject the null hypothesis. The investigator thus accepted by elimination the study hypothesis that an association exists between pipe smoking and mouth cancer in the general population.

Remember that we have defined *small* as a 5% chance or less that the observed results would have occurred if no true difference exists in the larger population. The 5% figure may be too large or too small if important decisions depend on the results. The 5% figure is based on some convenient statistical properties; however, it is not a magic number. It is possible to define *small* as 1%, 0.1%, or as any other probability one chooses. Remember, however, that no matter what

TABLE 5-1. HOW A STATISTICAL SIGNIFICANCE TEST WORKS

1. *State hypothesis*
   Develop the study question: An association exists between factors or a difference exists between groups in the general population.
2. *Formulate null hypothesis*
   Reverse the hypothesis: No association between factors or difference between groups exists in the general population.
3. *Decide significance level*
   ≤5% unless otherwise indicated and justified
4. *Collect data*
   Determine whether an association between factors or a difference between groups exists in the data collected from samples of the larger population.
5. *Apply statistical significance test*
   Determine the probability of obtaining the observed data if the null hypothesis were true (i.e., choose and apply the correct statistical significance test).
6. *Reject or fail to reject the null hypothesis*
   Reject the null hypothesis and accept by elimination the study hypothesis if the statistical significance level is reached. Fail to reject the null hypothesis if the observed data have more than a 5% probability of occurring by chance if there is no association between factors or difference between groups in the larger population.

level is chosen, there will always be some probability of rejecting the null hypothesis when no true difference exists. Statistical significance tests can measure this probability but they cannot eliminate it.

Table 5-1 reviews and summarizes the steps in performing a statistical significance test.

ERRORS IN STATISTICAL SIGNIFICANCE TESTING

Several types of errors commonly occur in using statistical significance tests:

1. Failure to state the hypothesis before conducting the study
2. Failure to correctly interpret the results of statistical significance tests by not considering the Type I error
3. Failure to correctly interpret the results of statistical significance tests by not considering the Type II error

Let us begin by observing the consequences of failure to state the hypothesis before conducting the study:

An investigator randomly selected 100 individuals known to have essential hypertension and 100 individuals known to be free of hypertension. He compared them according to a list of 100 variables to determine how the two groups differed. Of the 100 variables studied, two were found to be statistically significant at the 0.05 level using standard statistical methods: (1) hypertensives generally have more letters in their last name than nonhypertensives, and (2) hypertensives generally are born during the first $3^1/2$ days of the week whereas nonhypertensives are usually born during the latter $3^1/2$ days of the week. The author concluded that, despite the fact that these differences had not been foreseen, longer names and a birth during the first half of the week are statistically associated with essential hypertension.

This example illustrates the importance of stating the hypothesis beforehand. Whenever a large number of variables are tested, it is likely by chance alone that some of them will be statistically significant variables. If no hypothesis is stated beforehand, there can be no null hypothesis to reject. In addition, it can be misleading to apply the usual levels of statistical significance unless the hypothesis has been stated before collecting and analyzing the data. If associations are looked for only after collecting the data, much stricter criteria may be applied than the usual 5% probability.

When a single hypothesis is not stated, a suggested rule of thumb for the reader of the medical literature is to divide the observed P value by the number of variables being studied. The resulting P value can then be used to reject or fail to reject the null hypothesis. For instance, imagine that a study looked at five variables in each of two groups without stating a study hypothesis. To declare statistical significance for any one variable the P value for that variable must be equal to*

$$\frac{0.05}{\text{Number of variables}} = \frac{0.05}{5} = 0.01$$

This P value of 0.01 should be interpreted the same way one would interpret a P value of 0.05 if one study hypothesis were stated before beginning the study.†

This approach reduces the statistical power of a study to demonstrate statistical significance for any one variable. Thus many biostatisticians argue it is better to use the multivariable method, which will be discussed in *Part 4, Selecting a Statistic.*

---

* If there are more than two groups, the equation is the desired Type I error divided by the number of comparisons.

† This method is a useful approximation for small numbers of variables. As the number of variables increases much above 5, it tends to require too small a P value before declaring statistical significance.

Remember that statistical significance testing or hypothesis testing is a method of drawing inferences in a world in which we must decide between the study and the null hypothesis based *only on the data within the study.* * It is possible, however, to look at inference as a process that incorporates a probability that the hypothesis is true. In this process the investigator must estimate the probability that the hypothesis is true before the study begins. This might be done based on the results of previous studies or other medical knowledge. When this prior probability is obtained, statistical methods are available to estimate the probability that the hypothesis is true after the results of the study are obtained. This *Bayesian* process is parallel to the use of diagnostic testing, which we will discuss in *Part 2, Testing a Test.* An advantage of the Bayesian approach is that P values need not be adjusted to account for the number of variables.

Type I Errors

Some errors are inherent in the method of statistical significance testing. Fundamental to the concept of statistical significance testing is the possibility that a null hypothesis will be falsely rejected and a study hypothesis will be falsely accepted. This is known as a *Type I* error. In traditional significance testing, as much as a 5% chance of incorrectly accepting a study hypothesis exists even when no true difference exists in the larger population from which the study samples were obtained. This level of Type I error is known as the alpha level. Statistical significance testing does not eliminate uncertainty. Careful readers of studies are therefore able to appreciate the degree of doubt that exists and can decide for themselves whether they are willing to tolerate or act with that degree of uncertainty.

In some circumstances an alpha level of 0.05 may be more than one is willing to tolerate; in other circumstances one may tolerate even more than 5% uncertainty. For instance, before introducing a new method of water purification into a community with a low frequency of water-borne infection, one might not accept the conclusion if there is 5% probability that the new method would fail to kill disease organisms. On the other hand, in a community where water was a major

---

* It is possible to indirectly incorporate outside information into the statistical significance method by choosing the P value that will be used to declare statistical significance. For instance, when using a one-tailed statistical significance test, one is implying that previous data already imply that the hypothesis is true and the study is being conducted to determine the strength of the relationship. This approach, however, incorporates far less outside information than is possible using the Bayesian method.

source of disease transmission, one might tolerate a higher probability that the new method would fail to thoroughly eliminate water-borne disease, especially if no other method were available. Let us see how failure to appreciate the possibility of a Type I error can lead to misinterpretation of study results.

The author of a medical review article evaluated 20 well-conducted studies that examined the relationship between breast-feeding and breast cancer. Nineteen of the studies found no association between breast-feeding and breast cancer. One study found an association between breast-feeding and increased breast cancer significant at the 0.05 level. The author of the review article concluded that, since a study existed suggesting that breast-feeding is associated with an increased risk of breast cancer, breast-feeding should be discouraged.

When 20 well-conducted studies are performed to test an association that in fact does not exist, a substantial possibility exists that one of the studies may show an association at the 0.05 level simply by chance. Remember the meaning of statistical significance at the 0.05 level: It implies that the results have a 5% probability, or a chance of 1 out of 20, of occurring by chance alone when no association exists in the larger population. Thus 1 study in 20 that shows an association should not be interpreted as evidence for an association. It is important to keep in mind the possibility that no association may exist even when statistically significant results have been demonstrated. If the only study showing a relationship had been adopted without further questioning, breast-feeding might have been discouraged without producing any cancer prevention benefits.

Type II Errors

A *Type II* error says that failure to reject the null hypothesis does not necessarily mean that no true difference exists. Remember that statistical significance testing directly addresses only the null hypothesis. The process of statistical significance testing allows one to reject or not to reject that null hypothesis. It does not allow one to support a null hypothesis. Failure to reject a null hypothesis merely implies that the evidence is not strong enough to reject the assumption that no difference between groups or association between factors exists in the larger population.

Two factors may prevent an investigator from demonstrating a statistically significant difference even when one exists. Chance alone may produce an unusual set of data that fail to show a substantial difference even though one actually exists in the larger population. This type of error is parallel to a Type I error, indicating that chance has played a part. A particular study may come up with an unusual outcome that could occur only a small percentage of the time. It does not imply that mistakes were made in design or interpretation of the study; it merely points out that, despite the best efforts and intentions, statistical methods by the luck of the draw can produce incorrect conclusions. This factor is inherent in statistical concepts: Efforts to perform statistical significance testing always carry with them the probability of error.

Investigators may stack the odds against themselves by using too few individuals in a study. The fewer the number of individuals included in a study, the greater the impact of the chance occurrence of a few unusual individuals. The inclusion of unusual observations makes it more difficult to reject the null hypothesis. The fewer the number of individuals included in a study, the greater the true difference must be on average before statistically significant results can be demonstrated.

Conversely, the greater the number of individuals who are included in a study, the smaller the size of the true difference that can be demonstrated by the data to be statistically significant. At its extreme, this concept holds that any true difference, no matter how small, can be shown to be statistically significant if a great enough number of individuals are used in the study.

Statistical techniques are available for estimating the probability that a study could establish a statistically significant difference if a specified size-true difference actually exists in the larger population. These techniques measure the statistical "power" of the study. In many studies the probability is quite great that one will fail to show a statistically significant difference when a true difference actually exists. No arbitrary number indicates how great a Type II error one should tolerate. Without actually stating it, investigators who use relatively small samples may be accepting a 20%, 30%, or even greater risk that they will fail to demonstrate a statistically significant difference even when a true difference exists in the larger populations. Table 5-2 summarizes and compares Type I and Type II errors.

The following example shows the effect of sample size on the ability to demonstrate statistically significant differences between groups:

A study of the adverse effects of cigarettes on health was undertaken by following 100 cigarette smokers and 100 nonsmokers for 20 years. During the 20 years, five smokers developed lung cancer while none of the nonsmokers were afflicted. During the same time period, 10 smokers and 9 nonsmokers developed myocardial infarction. The results for lung cancer were statistically significant, but the results for myocardial infarction were not. The authors concluded that an association between cigarettes and lung cancer had been supported, and an

TABLE 5-2. INHERENT ERRORS OF STATISTICAL SIGNIFICANCE TESTING

	Type I error	Type II error
Definition:	Rejection of null hypothesis when no true difference exists in the larger population	Failure to reject null hypothesis when a true difference exists in the larger population
Cause:	Chance	Chance or a too small sample size
Likelihood of occurrence:	Setting of significance level will indicate how large an error will be tolerated (usually 5%)	Statistical techniques can estimate occurrence from the size of the groups (probability of error may be quite large if the numbers are small)

association between cigarette smoking and myocardial infarction had been refuted.

When differences between groups are very great, as they are between smokers and nonsmokers in relation to lung cancer, only a relatively small sample may be required to demonstrate statistical significance. When the true differences are smaller, it requires greater numbers to demonstrate a statistically significant difference. This study cannot be said to refute an association between cigarettes and myocardial infarction. It is very likely that the numbers used were too few to give the study enough statistical power to demonstrate an association between cigarettes and myocardial infarction even though other studies suggest that an association exists in the general population. A study with limited statistical power to demonstrate a difference also has limited power to refute a difference.

ADJUSTMENT

It was pointed out in Chapter 3 that the investigator is obligated to compare the individual characteristics of the study group with those of the control group to determine whether they differ in any way. If the groups differ, even without being statistically significant, the investigator must consider whether these differences could have affected the results. Characteristics that show differences between groups that may affect the results of the study are potential confounding variables. These potential confounding variables may result either from selection bias in case-control or cohort studies or from chance differences in all three of our basic types of studies. If a potential confounding variable is detected, the investigator is obligated to take this into consideration in the analysis with a process known as *adjustment of data.* *

In performing an adjustment, the investigator may separate into groups those who possessed various levels of the confounding variable. Groups with the same level of confounding variable are then compared to see if an association between exposure and disease exists. For instance, if age is a potential confounding variable, the investigator might subdivide the groups by age into several categories; the study and control groups in each age classification can then be compared to determine whether differences exist when the groups of similar age are compared. Statistical techniques known as *multivariable methods* are available for adjusting one or more variables at a time, as we discuss in Chapter 29. Failure to recognize and adjust for a confounding variable can result in serious errors as illustrated in the following example:

An investigator studied the relationship between coffee consumption and lung cancer by following 500 heavy coffee drinkers and 500 noncoffee drinkers for 10 years. In this cohort study, the risk for lung cancer in heavy coffee drinkers was 10 times that of coffee abstainers. The author concluded that coffee, along with cigarettes, was established as a risk factor in the development of lung cancer.

Cigarette smoking may be considered a confounding variable in this study if it is assumed that cigarette smoking is associated with coffee drinkers. In other words, coffee drinkers are more likely than noncoffee drinkers to smoke cigarettes. Furthermore, cigarettes are associated with lung cancer. Thus, cigarettes are a potential confounding factor related both to the outcome of lung cancer and to cigarette smoking. Figure 5-1 depicts the relationship between coffee drinking, cigarette smoking, and lung cancer. If cigarette smoking is a confounding variable, adjustment for cigarettes must be performed as part of the analysis.

In adjusting for cigarette smoking, the investigator would divide coffee drinkers into cigarette smokers and nonsmokers, and would do the same with the noncoffee drinkers. The investigator would then compare nonsmoking coffee drinkers with nonsmoking noncoffee drinkers to determine if the relationship between coffee drinkers and lung cancer still holds true. Only after determining that adjustment for cigarette smoking does not eliminate the relationship between coffee drinking and lung cancer can the author conclude that coffee drinking is associated with the development of lung cancer.

---

* Many biostatisticians encourage the use of adjustment, even when differences are not apparent, because of the possibility of interactions between variables.

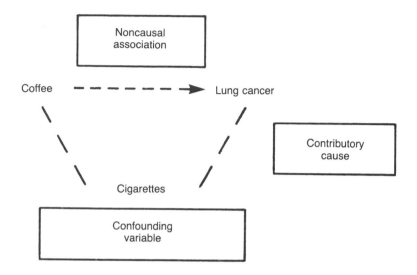

FIGURE 5-1   *Relationship between contributory cause, confounding variable, and noncausal association.*

STRENGTH OF RELATIONSHIP

Having examined the use of statistical methods to take confounding variables into account and to perform statistical significance testing, let us turn our attention to how statistical methods help us measure the strength of an observed association. First, we will look at the basic measure of the strength of an association that is most frequently used in cohort studies. Then we will turn to the basic measure used in case-control studies. Remember, by *association* we mean that a factor, often called a *risk* factor, occurs together with a disease more frequently than expected by chance alone. Notice that *association* does not necessarily imply a cause and effect relationship as we will examine in more detail in Chapter 6.

Let us assume that we are studying the association between birth control pills and thrombophlebitis. We want to measure the strength of the association to determine how the use of birth control pills affects the risk of developing thrombophlebitis. Therefore first we must clarify the concept of *risk*.

Risk measures the probability of developing a condition over a specified period of time. Risk equals the number of individuals who develop the condition divided by the number of individuals who were available to develop the condition at the beginning of the period. In assessing the 10-year risk of developing thrombophlebitis, we would divide the number of women on birth control pills who develop thrombophlebitis over a 10-year period by the total number of study group women on birth control pills without thrombophlebitis at the beginning of the study period.

A further calculation is necessary in order to measure the relative degree of association between thrombophlebitis for women who are on birth control pills compared to women who are not on birth control pills. One such measure is known as *relative risk*. Relative risk measures the risk of thrombophlebitis if birth control pills are used versus the risk if birth control pills are not used. It is defined as follows:

$$\text{Relative risk} = \frac{\text{Risk of developing thrombophlebitis if birth control pills are used}}{\text{Risk of developing thrombophlebitis if birth control pills are not used}}$$

generally,

$$\text{Relative risk} = \frac{\text{Risk of the outcome if the risk factor is present}}{\text{Risk of the outcome if the risk factor is absent}}$$

Let us illustrate how the risk and relative risk are calculated using a hypothetical example.

For 10 years an investigator followed 1,000 randomly selected young women on birth control pills and 1,000 randomly selected young women who were nonusers. He found that 30 of the women on birth control pills developed thrombophlebitis over the 10-year period while only 3 of the nonusers developed thrombophlebitis over the same time period. He presented his data using the following 2 × 2 table:

	THROMBOPHLEBITIS	NO THROMBOPHLEBITIS	
Birth control pills	a = 30	b = 970	a + b = 1,000
No birth control pills	c = 3	d = 997	c + d = 1,000

The 10-year risk of developing thrombophlebitis on birth control pills equals the number of women on the pill who develop thrombophlebitis divided by the total number of women on the pill. Thus,

Risk of developing thrombophlebitis for women on birth control pills

$$= \frac{a}{a + b} = \frac{30}{1,000} = 0.03$$

Likewise the 10-year risk of developing thrombophlebitis for women not on the pill equals the number of women not on the pill who develop thrombophlebitis divided by the total number of women not on the pill. Thus,

Risk of developing thrombophlebitis for women not on the pill

$$= \frac{c}{c + d} = \frac{3}{1,000} = 0.003$$

The relative risk equals the ratio of these two risks, thus,

$$\text{Relative risk} = \frac{a/a + b}{c/c + d} = \frac{0.03}{0.003} = 10$$

A relative risk of 1 implies that the use of birth control pills does not increase the risk of thrombophlebitis. This relative risk of 10 implies that, on the average, women on the pill have a risk of thrombophlebitis 10 times that of women not on the pill.

Now let us look at how we measure the strength of association for retrospective or case-control studies by looking at a study of the association between birth control pills and thrombophlebitis.

An investigator selected 100 young women with thrombophlebitis and 100 young women without thrombophlebitis. She carefully obtained the history of prior use of birth control pills. She found that 90 of the 100 women with thrombophlebitis were using birth control pills compared with 45 of the women without thrombophlebitis. She represented her data using the following 2 × 2 table:

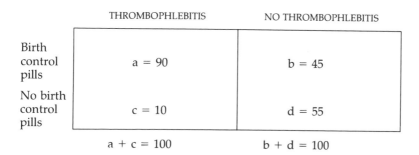

	THROMBOPHLEBITIS	NO THROMBOPHLEBITIS
Birth control pills	a = 90	b = 45
No birth control pills	c = 10	d = 55
	a + c = 100	b + d = 100

Notice that in case-control studies, the investigator can choose the total number of patients in each group (with and without thrombophlebitis). She could have chosen to select 200 patients with thrombophlebitis and 100 patients without thrombophlebitis or a number of other combinations. Thus the actual numbers in each vertical column can be altered at will by the investigator. In other words, in a case-control study the number of individuals who have and do not have the disease does not necessarily reflect the natural frequency of the disease. It is therefore improper to add the boxes horizontally in a case-control study (as we did in the preceding cohort study). In a case-control study this would allow the investigator to manipulate the size of the resulting relative risk.

Unfortunately, without numbers in the far right-hand side of the 2 × 2 table it is not possible to calculate risk as we did for the cohort study. However, a good approximation of relative risk exists for case-control studies, which turns out to be very useful for statistical analysis. This approximation of relative risk is known as the *odds ratio*.

First, what do we mean by *odds*, and how does that differ from probability or risk? Risk is a probability measure in which the numerator contains the number of times the event such as thrombophlebitis occurs over a specified period of time. The denominator of a risk of probability contains the number of times the event could have occurred. Odds, like probability, contain the number of times the event occurred in the numerator. However, in the denominator, odds contain the *number of times the event did not occur*. The difference between odds and probability may be appreciated by thinking of the chan·˙˙ of drawing an ace from a deck of 52 cards. The probability of drawing an ace is the number of times an ace will be drawn divided by the total number of cards or 4 out of 52 or 1 out of 13. Odds, on the other hand, are the number of times an ace will be drawn divided by the number of times it will not be drawn or 4 to 48 or 1 to 12. Thus, the odds are slightly different from the probability, but when the event or the disease under study is rare, the odds are a good approximation of the risk or probability.

The odds ratio measures the odds of having the risk factor if the condition is present divided by the odds of having the risk factor if the condition is not present. The odds of being on the pill if thrombophlebitis is present are equal to:

$$\frac{a}{c} = \frac{90}{10} = 9$$

Likewise, the odds of being on the pill for women who do not develop thrombophlebitis are measured by taking the number of women who do not have thrombophlebitis and are using the pill divided by the number of women who do not develop thrombophlebitis and are not on the pill. Thus, the odds of being on the pill if thrombophlebitis is not present are equal to

$$\frac{b}{d} = \frac{45}{55} = 0.82$$

Parallel with the calculation of relative risk, one can develop a measure of the relative odds of being on the pill if thrombophlebitis is present versus being on the pill if thrombophlebitis is not present. This measure of the strength of association is known as the odds ratio. Thus,

$$\text{Odds ratio} = \frac{\text{Odds of being on the pill if thrombophlebitis is present}}{\text{Odds of being on the pill if thrombophlebitis is not present}} = \frac{a/c}{b/d} = \frac{ad}{cb} = \frac{9}{0.82} = 11$$

An odds ratio of 1, parallel with our interpretation of relative risk, means that there are the same odds of being on the pill if thrombophlebitis is present compared with the odds of being on the pill if thrombophlebitis is absent. Our odds ratio of 11 means that the odds of being on birth control pills are increased 11-fold for women with thrombophlebitis.

The odds ratio serves as the basic measure of the degree of association for case-control studies. It is in and of itself a useful and valid measure of the strength of the association. In addition, as long as the disease (thrombophlebitis) is rare, the odds ratio approximates the relative risk.

It is possible to look at the odds ratio in reverse as one would do in a cohort study and come up with the same result. For instance,

$$\text{Odds ratio} = \frac{\text{Odds of developing thrombophlebitis if pill is used}}{\text{Odds of developing thrombophlebitis if pill is not used}}$$

The odds ratio then equals

$$\frac{\frac{a}{b}}{\frac{c}{d}} = \frac{ad}{cb} = 11$$

Notice that this is the same formula for the odds ratio as the one shown previously. This convenient property allows one to calculate an odds ratio from a cohort or controlled clinical trial instead of using the relative risk and to compare it directly to the odds ratio produced by a case-control study.

Thus relative risks and odds ratios are the fundamental measures we use to quantitate the strength of an association between a risk factor and a disease.

CONFIDENCE INTERVALS

When we discussed statistical significance testing we indicated that it does not provide information about the strength of an observed association. It is attractive to use a method that will provide a summary measure, often called a point estimate, of the strength of an association and also permits us to calculate a statistical significance test.

Confidence intervals are such a method of combining information from samples about the strength of an association with information about the effects of chance on the likelihood of obtaining the observed results. It is possible to calculate the confidence interval for any percentage confidence from 0 to 100. However, the 95% confidence interval is the most commonly used.

The 95% confidence interval allows us to be 95% "confident" that a large population's numerical value lies within the confidence interval.

Confidence intervals are often calculated for odds ratios and relative risks. The calculation of these intervals is complex. The reader of the literature, however, may see an expression such as 10(8,12), which expresses the odds ratio (lower confidence limit, upper confidence limit).

The term *confidence limit* is used to indicate the upper or lower extent of a confidence interval. This expression usually tells us the observed odds ratio and the 95% confidence interval. Other confidence intervals may be used, but they should be specifically indicated.

Imagine a study in which the odds ratio for birth control pills and thrombophlebitis was 10(8,12). How would you interpret this confidence interval?

The confidence interval on this odds ratio allows us to say with 95% confidence that the odds ratio in the larger population is between 12 and 8. This allows us to be quite confident that a substantial odds ratio is present not only in our sample but in the larger population from which our sample was obtained.

These expressions of confidence limits have another advantage for the reader of the clinical literature: They allow us to do hypothesis testing and rapidly draw conclusions about the statistical significance of the observed data. When using 95% confidence intervals, we can rapidly conclude whether or not the observed data are statistically significant with a P value less than or equal to 0.05.

This calculation is particularly simple for odds ratios and relative risks. For odds ratios and relative risks, 1 represents the point at which the odds or risk of disease are the same whether or not the risk factor is present. Thus an odds ratio of 1 is really an expression of the null hypothesis that says the odds of disease are the same if the risk factor is present and if it is absent.

Thus if the 95% confidence interval around the observed odds ratio fails to extend beyond or overlap 1, it is accurate to conclude that the odds ratio is statistically significant with a P value less than or equal to 0.05. The same principles are true for relative risks. Let us look at the following odds ratios and confidence intervals:

A. 4(0.9–7.1)
B. 4(2–6)
C. 8(1–15)
D. 8(6–10)
E. 0.8(0.5 1.1)
F. 0.8(0.7–0.9)

Since an odds ratio is statistically significant if the 95% confidence interval fails to extend beyond 1, examples B, C, D, and F are statistically significant with a P value less than or equal to 0.05, whereas examples A and E are not statistically significant since they have a P value greater than 0.05.

As a reader of the clinical literature, you will increasingly find the observed value and the confidence limits included in the analysis section. This is helpful because it allows you to gain a "gestalt" or a feel for the data. It allows you to draw your own conclusion about the clinical importance of size or strength of the observed point estimate. Finally for those who wish to convert to the traditional statistical significance testing format for hypothesis testing, one can often make an approximate calculation to determine whether the results are statistically significant with a P value of 0.05 or less.

CHAPTER 6

Interpretation

STATISTICALLY SIGNIFICANT VERSUS CLINICAL IMPORTANCE

Statistical significance testing is designed to help us assess the role of chance when we observe a difference or an association in an investigation. As we have discussed, statistical significance testing tells us very little about the size of a difference or the strength of an association. Thus it is important to ask not only is a difference or association statistically significant, but is it large or substantial enough to be clinically useful. The world is full of a myriad of differences between individuals and between groups. Many of these, however, are not great enough to allow us to usefully separate individuals into groups for purposes of diagnosis and therapy.*

As we have seen, when the sample size of a study is small, the possibility of a Type II error can be very great. Remember a Type II error is the probability of failing to demonstrate statistical significance when a true difference or association exists. Conversely when the sample size is quite large, it is quite possible to obtain a statistically significant difference or association even when the difference or association is too small or too weak to be clinically useful as in the following example:

---

* It is sometimes necessary to distinguish between statistically significant, substantial, and clinically important. At times statistically significant and large differences between groups are not useful for decision making. We may decide medically or socially to treat individuals the same regardless of large differences in such factors as intelligence, height, or age.

Investigators followed 100,000 middle-aged men for 10 years to determine which factors were associated with coronary artery disease. They hypothesized beforehand that uric acid might be a factor in predicting the disease. The investigators found that men who developed coronary artery disease had a uric acid measure of 7.8 mg/dl whereas men who did not develop the disease had an average uric acid measure of 7.7 mg/dl. The difference was statistically significant at the 0.05 level. The authors concluded that, since a statistically significant difference had been found, the results would be clinically useful.

The differences in the above study are statistically significant, but they are so small that they probably are not important clinically. The great number of men under observation allowed investigators to detect a very small difference between groups. However, the small size of the difference makes it unlikely that uric acid measurements could be clinically useful in predicting who will develop coronary artery disease. The small difference does not help the clinician to differentiate those who will develop coronary artery disease from those who will not. In fact, when the test is performed in the clinical laboratory, this small difference is probably less than the size of the laboratory error in measuring uric acid.

CONTRIBUTORY CAUSE

Can cigarettes cause cancer? Can cholesterol cause coronary artery disease? Can chemicals cause congenital defects? The clinician is constantly confronted with controversies over cause and effect. Thus the reader of the medical literature must have an understanding of the concept of causation used by investigators.

A practical clinical concept of causation is called *contributory cause*. It is an empirical definition that requires the fulfillment of the following criteria: (1) The characteristic referred to as the "cause" is associated with the disease (effect), that is, it occurs in the same individual as the disease more often than expected by chance alone; (2) Cause has been shown to precede the effect, that is, the cause acts at a time before the disease has developed; and (3) Altering only the cause has been shown to alter the probability of the effect (disease). The process of analysis including statistical significance testing and adjustment helps determine whether an association exists and whether it is produced by known biases. However, to establish the second and third criteria, we must rely on more than statistical analysis. It may appear simple to establish that a cause precedes a disease, but let us look at two hypothetical studies in which the authors may have been fooled into believing that they had established that cause precedes effect.

Two investigators, conducting a case-control study of drugs taken by patients with myocardial infarction (MI) the week preceding an MI, were looking for the precipitating causes of the condition. MI patients were compared with patients admitted for elective surgery. The authors found that the MI patients were 10 times as likely to have taken aspirin or antacids as the controls during the week preceding admission. The authors concluded that taking aspirin and antacids is associated with subsequent MIs.

The authors believed that they established not only the first criteria of causation (i.e., an association), but also the second criteria that the cause precedes the effect. But did they? If individuals have angina prior to MIs, they may misinterpret the pain and try to alleviate it by self-medicating with aspirin or antacids. Therefore, the medication is being taken to treat the disease and does not truly precede the disease. This study failed to establish that the "cause" precedes the "effect" because it did not clarify whether the disease led the patients to take the medication or whether the medication precipitated the disease. This example illustrates the potential difficulty encountered in separating cause and effect in case-control studies. Case-control studies, however, are often capable of providing convincing evidence that the "cause" precedes the "effect." This is the situation when there is good documentation of previous characteristics that are not affected by knowledge of occurrence of the disease.

Cohort or prospective studies often have an advantage in establishing that the possible cause occurs prior to the effect. The following example, however, illustrates that even in cohort studies we may have difficulty determining whether the cause precedes the effect.

A group of 1,000 patients who had stopped smoking cigarettes within the last year were compared to 1,000 current cigarette smokers matched for total-pack years of smoking. The two groups were followed for 6 months to determine the frequency with which they developed lung cancer. The study showed that 5% of the study group who had stopped smoking cigarettes developed lung cancer as opposed to only 0.1% of the controls. The authors concluded that to stop cigarette smoking was a prior characteristic associated with the development of lung cancer. Therefore, they advised current smokers to continue smoking.

The stopping of cigarette smoking appears to occur prior to the development of lung cancer, but what if smokers stop smoking because of symptoms produced by lung cancer? If this were true, then lung cancer stops smoking and not vice versa. Thus, one must be careful in accepting that the hypothesized cause precedes the effect. The ability of cohort studies to establish that the cause precedes the effect is enhanced when the time lapse between cause and effect is longer than in this example. Short time intervals still leave open the possibility that the cause has been influenced by the effect instead of the reverse.

Even if one has firmly established that the possible cause precedes the effect, it is necessary to establish that altering the cause alters the probability of the effect. This criterion can be established by performing an intervention study in which one alters the cause and determines whether this subsequently contributes to altering the probability of the effect. Ideally, this criterion is fulfilled by performing a controlled clinical trial as we will discuss in Chapter 11. It is important to recognize that contributory cause is an empirical definition. It does not require that we have an understanding of the intermediate mechanism by which the contributory cause brings about the effect. Historically, numerous instances occur in which actions based on a demonstration of contributory cause reduced disease despite the absence of a scientific understanding of how the result actually occurred. Puerperal fever was controlled through hand washing before the bacterial agents were recognized. Malaria was controlled by swamp clearance before its mosquito transmission was recognized. Scurvy was prevented by citrus fruit before the British ever heard of vitamin C. Figure 6-1 demonstrates the relationship between association, contributory cause, and direct and indirect cause.

Further investigations may be prompted by these studies that may establish the direct mechanism by which a contributory cause brings about its effect. Prior to understanding the immediate mechanism involved, the adoption of action based on this definition of cause and effect may well be warranted. Investigators, however, must be careful that any change that they have observed is not associated with other unmeasured changes that are the "real" contributory cause. This pitfall is illustrated by the following example:

In a poor rural community where the diet was very low in protein, diarrhea was widespread. The effect of increased protein was studied in randomly selected areas through the introduction of high-protein crops using modern agricultural methods. Subsequent follow-up revealed a 70% reduction in the incidence of diarrhea in the study areas with little change in the other areas. The authors concluded that a high-protein diet prevents diarrhea.

It is likely that the introduction of modern agriculture was associated with numerous other changes in water supply and sanitation that may have contributed as well to the reduced incidence of diarrhea. Thus, care must be taken to ensure that the characteristic selected as the cause is truly the factor that brought about the effect. In other words, the investigator and the reader must be careful that the cause has truly preceded the effect and that the presumed alter-

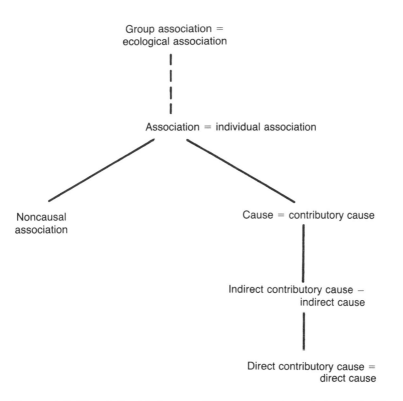

FIGURE 6-1 *The relationship between different types of associations and different definitions of causation.*

ation in the effect has not been produced by other changes that are actually causal. When contributory cause cannot be definitively established, we may still need to make our best judgments about the existence of a cause and effect relationship. For this situation a series of ancillary, adjunct, or supportive criteria for contributory cause have been developed. These include:

1. Strength of the association. The strength of the association between the risk factor and the disease as measured, for example, by the size of the relative risk.

2. The consistency of the association. Consistency is present when investigations performed in different settings on different types of patients produce similar results.

3. The biologic plausibility. The biologic plausibility of the relationship is evaluated based on clinical or basic science principles.

4. A dose-response relationship. A dose-response relationship implies that changes in levels of exposure to the risk factor are associated with changes in the frequency of disease in a consistent direction.

   Data that support each of these criteria help bolster the argument that a factor is actually a contributory cause. These criteria reduce the likelihood that the observed association is due to chance or bias. The criteria, however, do not prove the existence of a contributory cause. In addition, none of these four criteria for establishing contributory cause are essential. A risk factor with a modest but real association may in fact be one of a series of contributory causes for a disease. Consistency is not essential since it is possible for a risk factor to operate in one community but not in another. This may occur because of the existence in one community of other prerequisite conditions. Biological plausibility assumes that we understand the relevant biological processes. Finally a dose-response relationship, though frequent in medicine, is not required for a cause and effect relationship as illustrated in the next study.
   An investigator conducted a cohort study of the association between radiation and thyroid cancer. He found that low-dose radiation had a relative risk of 5 of being associated with thyroid cancer. However, he found that at moderate levels of radiation the relative risk was 10 and at high levels it was 1.0. The investigator concluded that radiation could not cause thyroid cancer since no dose-response relationship existed demonstrating more cancer with more radiation.
   The relative risk of 10 is an impressive association between radiation and thyroid cancer. This should not be dismissed merely because the relative risk is diminished at higher doses. It is possible that low-dose and moderate dose radiation contributes to thyroid cancer whereas large doses of radiation actually kill cells and thus do not contribute to thyroid cancer.
   Thus these ancillary, adjunct, or supportive criteria for judging contributory cause are just that: They do not in and of themselves settle the issue. They may, however, help support the argument for and against contributory cause. An appreciation of these criteria helps one understand the controversy and the limitations of the data.

OTHER CONCEPTS OF CAUSATION

The concept of contributory cause has been a very useful concept in studying disease causation. Contributory cause, however, is not the only concept of causation that has been used in clinical medicine. In the nineteenth century, Robert Koch developed a series of conditions that needed to be fulfilled before a microorganism could be considered the cause of a disease.* The conditions known as *Koch's postulates* include a requirement that the organism is always found with the disease. This condition is often called *necessary cause.*

Necessary cause goes beyond the requirements for establishing contributory cause. Historically, this was very useful in the study of infectious disease in circumstances where a single agent was responsible for a single disease. However, if the concept of necessary cause is applied to the study of chronic diseases, it is nearly impossible to prove a causal relationship. For instance, even though cigarettes have been well established as a contributory cause of lung cancer, cigarette smoking is not a necessary condition for the development of lung cancer; not all those with lung cancer have smoked cigarettes.

Under the rules of strict logic, causation also requires a second condition known as *sufficient cause.* This condition says that if the cause is present, so will be the disease. In our cigarette and lung cancer example sufficient cause would imply: if cigarette smoking is present lung cancer will always follow. To take another example, mononucleosis is a well-established clinical illness that has been shown to have the Epstein-Barr virus as a contributory cause. However, other viruses such as cytomegalovirus also have been shown to bring about the mononucleosis syndrome. In addition, Epstein-Barr virus may show evidence of having been present without ever causing the mononucleosis syndrome or it may manifest itself by being a contributory cause of other diseases such as Burkitt's lymphoma Thus, despite the fact that the Epstein-Barr virus has been established as a contributory cause of the mononucleosis syndrome, it is neither a necessary nor a sufficient cause of the mononucleosis syndrome. The next example illustrates the consequences of applying the necessary cause of formal logic to medical studies:

In a study of the risk factors for coronary artery disease, investigators identified 100 individuals from a population of 10,000 MI patients who experienced MIs despite normal blood pressure, normal cholesterol, regular exercise, no smoking, Type B personality, and no family history of coronary artery disease. The authors concluded that they had demonstrated that hypertension, high cholesterol, lack of exercise, smoking, Type A personality, and family history were not the causes of coronary artery disease since not every MI patient possessed a risk factor.

The authors of this study were using the concept of necessary cause as a concept of causation. Instead of necessary cause, however, let us assume that all these factors had been shown to fulfill the criteria

* Last, J. M. *A Dictionary of Epidemiology.* New York: Oxford University Press, 1988.

for contributory cause of coronary artery disease. Contributory cause, unlike necessary cause, does not require that all those who are free of the cause will be free of the effect. The failure of known contributory causes to predict all the cases of disease emphasizes the limitations of our current knowledge about all the contributory causes of coronary artery disease. It illustrates our current state of ignorance, for if all the contributory causes were known, then all those with disease would possess at least one such factor. Thus, even when a contributory cause has been established, it does not imply that it will necessarily be present in each and every case.

In summary, the clinically useful definition of causation is known as contributory cause. It requires a demonstration that the presumed cause precedes the effect, and that altering the cause alters the effect in some individuals. It does not require that all those who are free of the contributory cause will be free of the effect. It does not require that all those who possess the contributory cause will develop the effect. In other words, a clinically useful cause may be neither necessary nor sufficient, but it must be contributory. Its presence must increase the probability of the occurrence of disease and its absence must reduce the probability of the disease.

CHAPTER 7

Extrapolation

Previous chapters have illustrated the errors that can be made in assigning patients to study and control groups, assessing a study outcome, and analyzing and interpreting the results of a study. Having completed this process, the investigator now asks what meaning all this has for individuals not included in the study and for situations not directly addressed by the study. To obtain the meaning of the investigation for other groups or other situations, the investigator must extrapolate the results of the study to new and potentially different situations.* Let us start by seeing how we can use the outcome data of a study to extrapolate to similar individuals, similar groups at risk, and similar communities composed of individuals with and without the factors that have been studied. We will then explore extrapolation to new situations and new types of individuals

EXTRAPOLATION TO INDIVIDUALS

The first step in extrapolating the results of a study is to assess the overall meaning of the results for a particular individual, similar to those individuals included in the investigation. In doing this, we will assume that the finding in the study is as valid for other individuals with a risk factor being studied as it was for those individuals who were actually included in the investigation.

---

* One can argue that whenever data are used to draw conclusions about individuals who are not actually included in a study, extrapolation is occurring. In this situation we are extrapolating over time.

Many case-control and cohort studies estimate the odds ratios or relative risk associated with the development of the disease if a risk factor is present compared to when it is not present. Odds ratios and relative risks tell us the strength of the relationship between the risk factor and the disease. If a cause and effect relationship is present and the effect of the risk factor is completely reversible, the relative risks tell us important information for the individual patient. On average, a relative risk of 10 tells the individual patient that they will have 10 times the risk of developing the disease over a specified period of time if they have the risk factor compared to their risk if the risk factor is not present.*

However, relative risks do not tell us the absolute magnitude of the risk or the probability of developing the disease if the risk factor is present compared to when it is not present. A relative risk of 10 may indicate an increase in risk from 1 per 1,000,000 for those without the risk factor to 1 per 100,000 for those with the risk factor. Alternatively a relative risk of 10 may indicate an increase in risk from 1 per 100 for those without the risk factor to 1 per 10 among those with the risk factor. Thus despite the same relative risk, the absolute risk for individuals can be very different.

Failure to understand the concept of absolute risk can lead to the following type of extrapolation error:

A patient has read that the relative risk of leukemia is increased four times with use of a new chemotherapy for breast cancer; the relative risk of being cured of breast cancer by chemotherapy is 3. She therefore argues that the chemotherapy is not worth the risk.

The risk of dying from breast cancer, however, is far greater than the risk to the patient from leukemia. The infrequent and later occurrence of leukemia means that even in the presence of a risk factor that increases the risk fourfold, the absolute risk will still be very small compared to the very high risk of dying from breast cancer. The patient has failed to understand the important difference between relative risk and absolute risk. Thus it is desirable to have information on both the relative and absolute risk when extrapolating the results of a study to a particular individual.

EXTRAPOLATION TO AT-RISK GROUPS

Relative risk and absolute risk are often used to make estimates about individual patients. At times, however, we are more interested in the

* How well estimates of relative risk apply to an individual is actually determined by how similar the individuals included in the study are to the individual to whom we

effect that a risk factor may have on groups of individuals with the risk factor or on a community of individuals with and without the risk factor.

When assessing the effect of a risk factor on a group of individuals, we use a concept known as *attributable risk percentage.** Calculation of attributable risk percentage does not require existence of a cause and effect relationship. However, when a contributory cause exists, attributable risk percentage tells us the percentage of a disease that may be eliminated among those with the risk factor if the effects of the risk factor can be completely removed.†

Attributable risk percentage is defined as follows:

$$\frac{\text{Risk of disease if} \atop \text{risk factor present} - {\text{Risk of disease if} \atop \text{risk factor absent}}}{\text{Risk of disease if risk factor present}} \times 100\%$$

Attributable risk percentage can be more easily calculated from relative risk using the following formula:

$$\text{Attributable risk percentage} = \frac{\text{Relative risk} - 1}{\text{Relative risk}} \times 100\%$$

When the relative risk is less than 1

$$\text{Attributable risk percentage} = 1 - \text{Relative risk} \times 100\%$$

This is if

RELATIVE RISK	ATTRIBUTABLE RISK PERCENTAGE
1	0
2	50%
4	75%
10	90%
20	95%

Notice that even a relative risk of 2 may be associated with as much as a 50% reduction in the disease among those with the risk factor.

---

wish to apply the results. Application of results to an individual assumes that the study sample is composed entirely of persons exactly like that individual. It is not enough that persons like that individual are included in the study sample.
* Attributable risk percentage has also been called attributable fraction (exposed), etiological fraction (exposed), attributable proportion (exposed), percentage risk reduction, and protective efficacy rate.
† This interpretation of attributable risk requires that the effects of the risk factor can be immediately and completely removed.

Failure to understand this concept may lead to the following extrapolation error:

A large well-designed cohort study was conducted on men who exercised regularly versus men, matched for risk factors for coronary artery disease, who did not exercise regularly. The study found that those who did not exercise regularly had a relative risk of 1.5 of developing coronary artery disease. The investigators concluded that even if this were true, it was too small a relative risk to be of any practical importance.

Despite the fact that the relative risk is only 1.5, notice that it converts into a substantial attributable risk percentage.

$$\text{Attributable risk percentage} = \frac{1.5 - 1}{1.5} = \frac{0.5}{1.5} = 33\%$$

This says that among those who do not exercise regularly, a maximum of one-third of their risk could be eliminated if the effect of their lack of exercise could be eliminated. This may represent a large number of individuals since coronary artery disease is a frequently occurring disease and lack of regular exercise is a frequently occurring risk factor.

It can often be difficult to communicate the information contained in the absolute risk, relative risk, and attributable risk percentage. Another way of expressing this information, which is applicable to cohort studies and controlled clinical trials, is known as the *number needed to treat*.* The number needed to treat states the clinically important information: How many patients similar to the study patient need to be treated, as the average study group patient was, to obtain one fewer bad outcome or one more good outcome? The number is calculated as follows assuming that group A has a better outcome than group B:

$$\text{Number needed to treat} = \frac{1}{\text{Probability of the outcome in group A} - \text{Probability of the outcome in group B}}$$

Thus if an investigation demonstrated a reduction of coronary artery disease over a 5-year period from 20 per 1,000 to 10 per 1,000, the

---

* See Laupacis, A., Sackett, D. L., and Roberts, R. S. The assessment of clinically useful measures of the consequences of treatment. *N. Engl. J. Med.* 1988:1728–33.

number needed to treat for 5 years to obtain one less case of coronary artery disease would be calculated as follows:

$$\text{Number needed to treat} = \frac{1}{20/1{,}000 - 10/1{,}000}$$

$$= \frac{1}{10/1{,}000}$$

$$= 100$$

The number needed to treat often provides a more clinically useful means of discussing clinical research data than do the other summary statistics such as the relative risk of 2, or the attributable risk of 50%, or even the absolute risk of 20 per 1,000 versus 10 per 1,000.*

EXTRAPOLATION TO A COMMUNITY

When extrapolating the results of a study to a community of individuals with and without a risk factor, we need to use another measure of risk known as the *population attributable risk percentage (PAR)*.† The population attributable risk percentage tells us the percentage of the risk in a community that is associated with the exposure to a risk factor.‡ The calculation of population attributable risk percentage requires us to know more than the relative risk. It requires that we know or be able to estimate the percentage of individuals in the community who possess the risk factor. If we know the relative risk and percentage of individuals in the community with the risk factor (b) we can calculate population attributable risk percentage using the following formula:

$$\text{Population attributable risk percentage} = \frac{b\,(\text{Relative risk} - 1)}{b\,(\text{Relative risk} - 1) + 1} \times 100\%$$

This formula allows us to relate relative risk, b, and population attributable risk as follows:

* The number needed to treat can also be calculated for adverse effects. This allows a direct comparison between the number needed to prevent one adverse event and the number needed to treat to produce one side effect.
† Population attributable risk percentage has also been called attributable fraction (population), attributable proportion (population), and etiological fraction (population).
‡ This interpretation of PAR requires that a cause and effect relationship is present and that the consequences of the "cause" are immediately and completely reversible.

RELATIVE RISK	b	POPULATION ATTRIBUTABLE RISK (APPROXIMATE)
2	1%	1%
4	1%	3%
10	1%	8%
20	1%	16%
2	10%	9%
4	10%	23%
10	10%	46%
20	10%	65%
2	50%	33%
4	50%	60%
10	50%	82%
20	50%	90%
2	100%	50%
4	100%	70%
10	100%	90%
20	100%	95%

Notice that if the risk factor is uncommon (1% for instance), the relative risk must be substantial before the population attributable risk percentage becomes impressive. On the other hand, if the risk factor is common, 50% for instance, even a small relative risk means that the potential community impact may be substantial. When the prevalence of the risk factor is 100% (i.e., when everyone has the risk factor), notice that the population attributable risk percentage equals the attributable risk percentage.

Failure to understand the concept of population attributable risk can lead to the following extrapolation error:

Investigators report that a hereditary form of high cholesterol known as Type III hyperlipidemia occurs in 1 per 100,000 Americans. They also report that those with Type III hyperlipidemia have a relative risk of 20 of developing coronary artery disease. The authors concluded that a cure for Type III hyperlipidemia would have a substantial impact on the national problem of coronary artery disease.

Using the data and our formula for population attributable risk percentage, we find that elimination of coronary artery disease secondary to Type III hyperlipidemia produces a population attributable risk of about one fiftieth of 1%. Thus the fact that Type III hyperlipidemia is so rare a risk factor means that eliminating its impact cannot be expected to have a substantial impact on the overall occurrence of coronary artery disease.

EXTRAPOLATION TO NEW SITUATIONS

Extrapolation to new situations or different types of individuals is even more difficult and is often the most difficult step for the reader of research. It is difficult because the investigator and the reviewers are usually not able to adequately address the issues of interest to a particular reader. It is up to you, the reader. The investigator does not know your community or your patients. Despite the difficulty with extrapolating research data, it is impossible to practice medicine without extrapolation from clinical research. Often we must go beyond the data based on reasonable assumptions. If one is unwilling to do any extrapolation, then one is limited to applying research results to individuals who are nearly identical to those in a study.

Despite the importance of extrapolation, it is important to recognize the types of errors that can occur if extrapolation is not carefully performed. When extrapolating to different groups or different situations, two basic types of errors can occur: Errors may occur because of extrapolations beyond the data, and errors may occur due to the difference between the study group and the *target group,* the target group being the group about which we wish to draw conclusions.

BEYOND THE RANGE OF DATA

In clinical studies, individuals are usually exposed to the factors thought to be associated with the outcome for only a limited amount of time at a limited range of exposure. The investigators may be studying a factor such as hypertension that results in a stroke or a therapeutic agent such as an antibiotic that is associated with the cure of an infection. In either case, the interpretation must be limited to the range and duration of hypertension experienced by the subjects or the dosage and duration of the antibiotic employed in the study. When the investigators draw conclusions that go beyond the duration and range experienced by the study subjects, they frequently are making unwarranted assumptions. They may assume that longer exposure will continue to produce the same effect experienced by the study subjects. The following example illustrates a potential error resulting from extrapolating beyond the range of the data:

A new antihypertensive agent was tested on 100 resistant hypertensives. It was found to lower diastolic blood pressure in all 100 resistant hypertensives from 120 to 110 at doses of 1 mg per kg and from 110 to 100 at doses of 2 mg per kg. The authors concluded that this agent would be able to lower diastolic blood pressure from 100 to 90 at doses of 3 mg per kg.

It is possible that clinical evidence would document the new agent's efficacy at 3 mg per kg. Such documentation, however, awaits empirical proof. Many antihypertensive agents have been shown to reach maximum effectiveness at a certain dose and do not increase their effectiveness at higher doses. To conclude that higher doses produce greater effects without experimental evidence is to make a linear extrapolation beyond the range of the data.

Another type of error associated with extrapolation beyond the range of the data concerns potential side effects experienced at increased exposure, as can be seen in the following hypothetical example:

A 1-year study of the effects of administering daily unopposed estrogen to 100 menopausal women found that the drug relieved hot flashes and reduced the rate of osteoporosis as opposed to the lack of relief of symptoms in age-matched women given placebos. The authors found no adverse effects from the estrogens and concluded that estrogens are safe and effective. Therefore they recommended that unopposed estrogens be administered long-term to women, beginning at the onset of menopause.

The authors have extrapolated from a 1-year period of follow-up to long-term administration of unopposed estrogens. No evidence exists to show that if 1 year of administration is safe, so is long-term, continuous administration of unopposed estrogen. It is not likely that any long-term adverse effects would show up in a 1-year study. Thus, the authors have made potentially dangerous extrapolations by going beyond the range of their data.

Linear extrapolation may be necessary at times to the practice of medicine, but clinicians need to recognize that linear extrapolation has taken place so they can be on the lookout for new data that may undermine the assumptions and thus challenge the conclusion obtained by linear extrapolation.

DIFFERENCE IN THE TARGET GROUP

When extrapolating to a target group, it is important to consider how that group differs from the one in the investigation. The following scenario illustrates how differences between countries can complicate extrapolation from one country to another:

In a study of both Japanese society and American society, the Japanese were found to have a 20% prevalence of hypertension and an 80% prevalence of cigarette smoking, both known contributory causes of coronary artery disease among Americans. Americans were found to have a 10% prevalence of hypertension and a 40% prevalence of cigarette smoking. Case-control studies in Japan did not demonstrate an association between hypertension or cigarettes and coronary artery disease while similar studies in the United States demonstrated a statistically significant association. The authors concluded that hypertension and cigarette smoking must protect the Japanese from myocardial infarctions.

The authors have extrapolated from one culture to a very different culture. Other explanations for the observed data are possible. If Americans frequently possess another risk factor, such as high cholesterol, which is rare in Japan, this factor may override cigarette smoking and hypertension and help to produce the high rate of myocardial infarctions in the American population.

Extrapolation within countries can also be difficult when differences exist between the group that was investigated and the target group to which one wishes to apply the findings, as illustrated in the next example:

A study of the preventive effect of treating borderline tuberculosis (TB) skin tests (6–10 mm) with a year of isoniazid was conducted among Alaskan Eskimos. The population had a prevalence of borderline skin tests of 2 per 1,000. The study was conducted by giving isoniazid to 200 Eskimos with borderline skin tests and placebos to 200 other Eskimos with the same borderline condition. Twenty cases of active TB occurred among the placebo patients and only one among the patients given isoniazid. The results were statistically significant at the 0.05 level. A health official from Georgia, where borderline skin tests occur in 300 per 1,000 skin tests, was very impressed with these results. He advocated treating all patients in Georgia who had borderline skin tests with isoniazid for 1 year.

In extrapolating to the population of Georgia, the health official assumed that borderline skin tests meant the same among Alaskan Eskimos as among the population of Georgia. Other data suggest, however, that many borderline skin tests in Georgia are not due to TB exposure. Instead of indicating TB, they are frequently caused by an atypical mycobacteria that carries a much more benign prognosis and does not reliably respond to isoniazid. The health official ignored the fact that borderline skin tests have a very different meaning among Eskimos compared with residents of Georgia. By not appreciating this new factor in the residents of Georgia, the health official may be submitting large numbers of individuals to useless and potentially dangerous therapy.

Extrapolation of study results is always a difficult but extremely important part of reading the medical literature. Extrapolation involves first asking what the results mean for individuals like the average individual included in the investigation. Then one can ask what the results mean for similar at-risk groups and finally communities composed of individuals with and without the characteristics under study. Often the reader will want to go one step furthur and extend the extrapolation to individuals and situations that are different from those in the study. This extrapolation beyond the data must take into account the differences between the types of individuals included in the investigation and the target group. Recognizing the assumptions we make in extrapolation forces us to keep our eyes open for new information that challenges these assumptions and potentially invalidates our conclusions.

CHAPTER 8

Study Design

Since our discussion of the requirements for proper implementation of the components of the uniform framework is complete, let us go back to the beginning and ask some basic questions.

1. Were the aims of the study adequately defined?
2. What is the study type? Is it appropriate to the questions being asked?
3. How big is the study sample? Is it adequate to answer the study questions?

The answers to these questions will tell the reader whether the investigators have chosen an appropriate study design, that is, one that defines and addresses the intended study questions.

AIM OF THE STUDY

Investigators may desire to study the end-organ effects of hypertension, but the inability to perform renal biopsies and cerebral angiograms may force them to carefully study retinal changes. Researchers may wish to investigate the long-term effects of a new drug to prevent osteoporosis, but time, money, and the desire to publish may limit their investigation to its short-term effects on bone metabolism and bone density. It is essential that the investigators and the reader distinguish between what the investigators ideally would like to study and what they are in fact studying.

In further defining the aims of the study, a specific study hypothesis is essential. When studying end-organ damage due to hypertension, the investigators might hypothesize that the degree of end-organ damage will correlate with the degree of hypertension. This, however, is not specific enough to study. A specific hypothesis is required, such as: an increased degree of narrowing of the retinal arteries, as measured on retinal photographs after 3 years of observation, will correlate with an increased level of diastolic blood pressure taken as the average of three blood pressure measurements at the beginning of the study. The latter formulation provides a specific study question that can be addressed by an investigation.

Failure to clarify the hypotheses being tested makes it difficult for the researcher and for the reader to choose and assess the study design. It also makes it more difficult in the end to determine whether the aims of the study have been achieved. Finally, as was pointed out in our discussion of statistical significance testing, the usual tests of statistical significance are not applicable unless one defines a specific end point or outcome to be assessed.

EVALUATING THE STUDY TYPE

Having defined the specific study hypotheses, the reader is ready to identify the type of study that was performed and to evaluate the appropriateness of the type chosen. Rarely is only one type of study design appropriate to a study question. At times, however, the disadvantages of one type of study design may make it very difficult to accomplish the study aims. In order to help the reader judge the appropriateness of a chosen study design, let us outline the advantages and disadvantages of our basic types of studies.

Case-control or retrospective studies have the distinct advantage of being able to study rare conditions or diseases. If the condition is rare, case-control studies are able to detect differences between groups using far fewer individuals than would be required using other study designs. The time required to perform a case-control study is often much shorter, since the disease has already developed. The case-control method allows investigators to simultaneously explore the multiple possible associations with a disease. One could examine, for instance, the many variables that possibly are associated with colon cancer. Prior diet, surgery, ulcerative colitis, polyps, alcohol, cigarettes, family history, and many other variables all might be investigated in the same study.

The major objection to case-control studies is that they are prone to the variety of methodological errors and biases that were illustrated in the hypothetical studies. Many of the biases such as reporting and recall bias involve the accuracy of the data about prior characteristics. However, the case-control method may be an adequate method for establishing a prior association especially when there is no reason to believe that the researcher's or the study subject's knowledge of the presence of a disease affects the assessment of past data.

Cohort studies have the major advantage of greater assurance that the characteristic under study preceded the outcome under study. This is a critical distinction when assessing a cause and effect relationship. *Concurrent cohort* studies, which follow patients forward over long periods of time, are expensive and time-consuming. It is possible, however, to perform a cohort study without such a lengthy follow-up time. If reliable data on the presence or absence of the study characteristic are available from an earlier time, these data can be used to perform a *nonconcurrent cohort* study. In a nonconcurrent cohort study, the assignment of individuals to groups is made on the basis of this past data. After assignment has occurred the investigator can then look at the data on subsequent disease occurrence.

For instance, if cholesterol readings were available on a group of young adults from 15 years before the current study began, the patients who have not yet developed clinical consequence of high cholesterol could be followed forward in time to assess the subsequent development of coronary artery disease, strokes, or other consequences of high cholesterol that might occur soon after the time the study begins. The critical element, which characterizes all cohort studies, is the identification of individuals for study and control groups without knowledge of whether the disease or condition under study has developed.*

Cohort studies are able to delineate various types of consequences that are associated with a single risk factor. Researchers can simultaneously study the relationship between hypertension and stroke, myocardial infarction, heart failure, or renal disease. Cohort studies can produce more in-depth understanding of the effect of an etiological factor on multiple outcomes, but they are less likely than case-control studies to uncover new etiological factors.

Both case-control and cohort studies are observational; that is, they observe the characteristics and outcomes of individuals rather than impose the characteristics. Randomized clinical trials are distinguished from observational studies by the intervention that occurs

---

* Increasingly cohort studies are performed on large data bases that have already been completed before a study begins. This situation is the extreme of nonconcurrent study and is sometimes referred to as a *retrospective cohort study*. The key that makes these studies cohort studies is that the individuals are identified for inclusion in the study and control groups without knowledge of whether disease developed.

when an investigator randomizes individuals to study and control groups. The ability to assign individuals helps to ensure that the study characteristic and not some underlying predisposition produces the study results. When properly performed, randomized clinical trials are able to support all three criteria for contributory cause.

We will explore in-depth the strengths and weaknesses of controlled clinical trials in Chapters 11 and 12.

It may be helpful to review a possible sequence of studies conducted to establish the existence of a contributory cause. Researchers often begin with a case-control study when exploring for possible causes.* Case-control studies have the advantage of speed, low cost, and the ability to study numerous possible causes all at once. The case-control method aims to establish the existence of associations or relationships between factors. At times case-control studies can be relied on to assure us that the cause precedes the effect, but they may leave some doubt as to which comes first.

Once an association is established in one or more case-control studies, investigators frequently proceed to concurrent cohort studies. Despite the need for careful interpretation as illustrated in the smoking cessation example, the concurrent cohort method is often better able to establish that the cause precedes the effect.

After establishing that a possible cause precedes the effect, investigators might turn to an intervention study such as a randomized clinical trial to establish that altering the cause alters the effect. In a randomized clinical trial, individuals are randomized and blindly assigned to study or control groups. Only the study group is exposed to the possible cause or proposed treatment. The randomized clinical trial ideally establishes all three criteria of contributory cause and is thus a powerful tool for demonstrating contributory cause.

This sequence of studies might in theory proceed as follows: To establish that unopposed estrogen is a contributory cause of uterine cancer, an investigator might begin by conducting a case-control study exploring numerous variables, including a hypothesized association between unopposed estrogens and uterine cancer. If an association is found, the investigators might then conduct a concurrent cohort study to more firmly establish that taking estrogens precedes uterine cancer. They would want to be sure that estrogens are not given to treat any bleeding that could be a symptom of cancer. A concurrent cohort study would begin with similar groups of women who have been taking estrogen and not taking estrogen. Both groups

---

* With the increasing availability of large data bases investigators may begin by performing a nonconcurrent cohort study that also can be done quickly and at low cost.

would be followed over a period of time. The investigators would determine whether the estrogen-taking group develops more uterine cancer than the group not taking estrogen. This concurrent cohort study may more firmly establish that taking unopposed estrogens precedes the subsequent development of uterine cancer.

In theory, the investigation would then proceed with a controlled clinical trial randomizing women to unopposed estrogens or placebo. After providing suggestive evidence that unopposed estrogens are dangerous, however, it might be unethical or impractical to conduct a controlled clinical trial of the relationship between estrogens and uterine cancer. Investigators may then construct a *natural experiment* to provide support for the idea that estrogens are a contributory cause of uterine cancer. Such a natural experiment may occur, for instance, if one group discontinues estrogen use as a result of the publicity generated by the studies. If the group that discontinued estrogen use experiences a declining uterine cancer rate not found in a similar group that continues estrogen use, this natural experiment may provide the best available evidence that altering the cause alters the effect.

The basic types of studies discussed here are not the only types of studies one will encounter in the medical literature. Cross-sectional studies also are frequently performed. In these investigations the study characteristic and the outcome are measured at the same point in time; in other words, the assignment and assessment are performed at the same point in time. Cross-sectional studies are relatively rapid and inexpensive to perform. They are useful when one expects that exposure is not likely to change over time or that the time between exposure and disease is very short. When studying thrombophlebitis and its relationship to birth control pills, one might use a cross-sectional study. One would study whether women with thrombophlebitis are more likely to be on birth control pills at the time they develop thrombophlebitis.

SAMPLE SIZE

Having assessed the study aims and the study type, the reader should concentrate on the size of sample of individuals selected for study. The reader should ask this question: Are there an adequate number of patients to allow a reasonable chance of demonstrating a statistically significant difference between the study samples if a difference actually exists between the larger population from which the study samples are drawn?

In addressing the question of adequacy of sample size, we need to distinguish between case-control studies on the one hand, and cohort and randomized clinical trials on the other hand. Remember that in case-control studies, the outcome is a characteristic of the patient, whereas in cohort and randomized clinical trials the outcome is the disease. Thus in case-control studies of thrombophlebitis one would be interested in the size of a true difference in use of birth control pills which is likely to be shown to be statistically significant, given the sample size used in the study. In cohort or randomized clinical trials one is interested in how small a true difference in the probability of developing a disease such as thrombophlebitis is likely to be shown to be statistically significant, given the sample size used in the study.

Answers to these questions depend on the size of the Type I and Type II errors that the reader and investigator are willing to tolerate. Remember that a Type II error is the probability of failing to demonstrate a statistically significant difference when a true difference actually does exist in the larger populations from which the study and control groups are sampled.

The Type I error that will be tolerated is usually set at 5%. The Type II error that will be tolerated is open for discussion. Most investigators would like the probability of failing to demonstrate the statistical significance of a true difference to be 10% or less. If we assume a 5% Type I error and a 10% Type II error and apply standard statistical tables, then the following approximate sample size conclusion can be drawn:*

1. If 100 individuals will be included in the study group and 100 will be in the control group, an investigation has statistical power to demonstrate a statistically significant difference if the true frequency of an outcome such as death in one population is 20% or more and the true frequency of the outcome in the other population is 5% or less.
2. If the study group and the control group each will contain 250 individuals, then the investigation has statistical power to demonstrate a statistically significant difference if the true frequency of the outcome in one population is 20% or more and the true frequency of the outcome in the other population is 10% or less.
3. If the study group and the control group each will contain 500 individuals, then the investigation has statistical power to demonstrate statistical significance if the true frequency of the outcome in one population is 10% or more and the true frequency of outcome in the other population is 5% or less.

* Fleiss, J. L. *Statistical Methods for Rates and Proportions* (2nd ed.). New York: Wiley, 1981. Pp. 260–280.

4. When the frequency of both outcomes is low, and the percentage difference in outcomes is small, very large sample sizes are required to demonstrate statistical significance. For instance, to demonstrate statistical significance for true differences of 2% in one population and 1% in a second population, over 3,500 individuals are required in each group in the investigation. Remember when using these guidelines that even with very high statistical power a particular sample drawn from populations with a true difference may still fail to demonstrate statistical significance.

These ballpark estimates are useful for the reader of the literature since they allow the reader to gauge whether the study had a realistic prospect of demonstrating statistical significance given its sample size.

Let us now apply these principles of sample size to demonstrate why case-control studies are useful for studying rare diseases that affect relatively small numbers of individuals. Remember that the term *outcome* refers to a characteristic of a patient in case-control studies, and to the disease itself in cohort and randomized clinical trials. The following hypothetical study shows the difficulty in demonstrating statistical significance when a cohort study is used to investigate a rare disease:

Investigators wished to study whether birth control pills are associated with the rare occurrence of strokes in young women. The researchers followed 20,000 women on birth control pills and 20,000 women on other forms of birth control for 10 years. After spending millions of dollars in follow-up, they found two cases of stroke among the pill users and one case among the nonpill users. The differences were not statistically significant.

When a disease is very rare, such as strokes in young women, it often requires enormous numbers of individuals to demonstrate a statistically significant difference if a cohort study is used. Assume, for instance, that the rate of strokes among young women not on the pill is 1 per 100,000 or 0.001%. Let us further assume that birth control pills increase this risk 10-fold to 1 per 10,000 or 0.01%. The difference in outcome is thus 0.01% to 0.001% or 0.009%. The use of a cohort study to demonstrate a statistically significant difference for a true difference this small may require well over 100,000 women in each group.

On the other hand, if a case-control study is performed using young women with strokes as the study group and young women without strokes as the control group, the outcome being measured is now the use of birth control pills rather than strokes. Groups of 100 each will then be adequate for detecting a statistically significant difference if there actually is a difference in the use of birth control pills of 20% among women with strokes versus 5% of similar women without strokes. In this instance, it is feasible to perform a case-control study of the relationship between birth control pills and strokes, using only a small fraction of the individuals required to study the same question with a cohort study. Therefore this cohort study was doomed to failure from the beginning; a case control study would have been far more appropriate. Whenever an investigation fails to demonstrate a statistically significant difference, the reader must ask whether the study had adequate sample size to be able to produce statistically significant results.

In Chapter 11 we will explore in more depth the implications of sample size. Thus an evaluation of study design requires the reader to appreciate the aims of the study, the appropriateness of the study type being employed, and the adequacy of the sample size. Equipped with an understanding of these basic issues, the reader can evaluate the results of the study more intelligently.

CHAPTER 9

Summary: Studying a Study

STUDY DESIGN

In determining whether the study was properly designed to answer the study questions, the reviewer must initially determine whether the study aims were sufficiently defined and whether the study hypothesis was clearly delineated. Then the reader may need to ask whether the sample size was adequate to answer the study question.

The reader of the literature must also ask whether the study type employed was appropriate to the question being asked, taking into account the advantages and disadvantages of each type of study.

ASSIGNMENT

Investigators attempt to assemble study and control groups that are identical in all respects except for the characteristic(s) under study. Case-control and cohort studies are susceptible to *selection bias*. Selection bias occurs whenever study or control groups are chosen in such a way that they have different frequencies of a risk factor or prognostic factor that affects the outcome of the investigation. Selection bias is a special type of confounding variable produced by chance differences between the study and control groups that are related to the study outcome. When potential confounding variables occur, it is important that they be recognized so that they can be taken into account as part of the analysis.

ASSESSMENT

In assessing the outcome of a study, the reader must consider whether the requirements for a valid assessment have been fulfilled. The investigators must show that they have chosen an appropriate measure of outcome, one that measures what they intended to measure. They must have performed an accurate assessment, with a measurement that approximates the true measurement of the phenomenon. The measurement of outcome must be complete. Finally, they must have considered whether the process of observation affected the outcome being assessed.

ANALYSIS

Analysis involves the use of statistical methods to deal with the effects of chance, the effects of bias, and to make point estimates from sample data. Bias or chance may produce confounding variables that can be prevented at the beginning of the study by matching study and control groups or by pairing individuals in the study and control groups. Statistical significance testing procedures are methods of hypothesis testing that assess the effects of chance on the results of an investigation. Statistical significance testing often assumes one hypothesis and is prone to Type I and Type II errors. It involves a method of proof by elimination. In clinical studies, odds ratios and relative risks are basic measures of the strength of an association. The 95% confidence intervals are increasingly being substituted for or given as additional information. They provide the observed numerical value or point estimate as well as the range of values within which we can be 95% confident that the population's true value lies. Statistical significance testing and confidence intervals are derived using the same statistical methods. At times the reader of the medical literature can rapidly use confidence intervals to perform a statistical significance test.

INTERPRETATION

The authors of a study must ask what the results mean for persons included in the investigation. They must ask whether the size of the differences or strength of the association is such that the results are clinically useful or important. They must also ask whether the criteria for a cause and effect relationship have been established.

The authors and reader should apply the clinical concept of contributory cause. Contributory cause requires that the presumed cause is associated with and precedes the effect, and in addition, altering the cause alters the effect. It does not require that the cause is necessary or is sufficient to produce the effect. When the definite criteria cannot be established, ancillary adjunct or supportive criteria, including strength of the association, consistency of the association, biological plausibility, and the existence of a dose-response relationship, help support a judgment about the existence of a cause and effect relationship.

EXTRAPOLATION

Finally the reader must ask what the study results mean for those not included in the study. In extrapolating to an individual, the reader must distinguish between relative risk and absolute risk. When extrapolating to new groups with the risk factor, the number needed to treat provides a useful summary measure of the number of individuals who must be treated to obtain one fewer bad outcome or one more good outcome. We must also consider the attributable risk percentage. When extrapolating to populations composed of individuals with and without the risk factor, one must consider the population attributable risk percentage. One must recognize the danger of linear extrapolation beyond the range of the data. One must also consider how different characteristics of a new target population can affect the ability to extrapolate the results

Few investigations are free of all these errors; however, their presence does not automatically invalidate an investigation It is the responsibility of the careful reader to recognize the errors and take them into account when applying the results of the study.

QUESTIONS TO ASK IN STUDYING A STUDY

Let us now put the foregoing material together and see if you can apply what you have learned to simulated research articles. The critical method for evaluating a research study is outlined in the following checklist of questions to ask when you are studying a study:

1. Study design: Was the study properly designed?
   a. Were the aims of the study sufficiently defined? Were the study hypotheses clearly delineated?
   b. What was the study type? Was it appropriate to the questions being asked?

    c. How large were the study groups? Were they of adequate size to address the study questions?

2. Assignment: Was the assignment of patients to study and control groups proper?

    a. If the study was case-control or cohort, could selection bias have occurred?

    b. If the study was a randomized clinical trial, was randomization and blind assignment maintained?

    c. Regardless of the study type, were the study and control groups comparable with respect to characteristics other than the study factor(s), or could a confounding variable affect the results?

3. Assessment: Was the assessment of outcome properly performed in the study and the control groups?

    a. Was the measure of outcome appropriate to the study aims?

    b. Was the measure of outcome accurate, reflecting the true measurement of the phenomenon?

    c. Was the measure of outcome complete?

    d. Did the process of observation affect the outcome?

4. Analysis: Did the analysis properly compare the outcomes in the study and the control groups?

    a. Were the results adjusted to take into account the effect of possible confounding variables?

    b. Was a statistical significance test properly performed to assess the probability that the observed difference or association was due to chance if the null hypothesis were true?

    c. Was a point estimate and 95% confidence limit provided?

    d. Were the number of hypotheses taken into account? Alternatively, using a Bayesian approach was a prior probability placed on each hypothesis before the study began so that a probability of the hypotheses after the data were obtained could be calculated?

    e. Could a Type I or Type II error explain the study result?

5. Interpretation: Were valid conclusions drawn about the meaning of the investigation for those included in the study group?

    a. Is the size of the difference or strength of the association great enough to be clinically useful or important?

    b. Were all three criteria of contributory cause fulfilled?

    c. Did the investigators distinguish between contributory cause and necessary and sufficient cause?

    d. If all three criteria of contributory cause could not be fulfilled, were the ancillary criteria satisfied?

6. Extrapolation: Were the extrapolations to individuals and situations not included in the study properly performed?

a. Did the investigators consider both the relative risk and absolute risk when extrapolating to individuals?

b. When extrapolating to new groups with the risk factor, did the investigators take into account the attributable risk percentage?

c. When extrapolating to the new groups composed of individuals with and without the risk factor, did the authors take into account the population attributable risk percentage?

d. Did the authors perform a linear extrapolation beyond the data?

e. Did the authors consider differences between the study group and the target population?

CHAPTER 10

Flaw-Catching Exercises: Observational Studies

The following hypothetical studies include errors of the type illustrated in each of the components of the basic framework. These flaw-catching exercises are designed to test your ability to apply the basic framework in order to critically study a study. Examples of case-control and cohort studies are presented. Please read the exercises and write a critique of each study. A sample critique that points out important errors follows each exercise.

Note that the final flaw-catching exercise is the same one that you read at the beginning of the book. Compare your current critique of this review exercise to the one you wrote previously to see how much progress you have made.

EXERCISE NO. 1: CASE-CONTROL STUDY

A case-control study was undertaken in order to study the factors associated with the development of congenital heart disease (CHD) in fetuses. Two hundred women with first-trimester spontaneous abortions in which congenital heart abnormalities were found in the fetus on pathological examination were used as the study group. The control group was composed of 200 women with consecutive first-trimester–induced abortions in which no congenital heart defects were found.

An attempt was made to interview each one of the 400 women within 1 month after her abortion to determine which factors in the pregnancy may have led to CHD. One hundred different variables were studied. The interviewers gained the participation of 120 of the 200 study group women who experienced spontaneous abortions and 80 of the 200 control group women who underwent induced abortions. The other women refused to participate in the study.

The investigators found the following differences between women whose fetuses had CHD and those whose fetuses were not affected:

1. Women with CHD fetuses were three times as likely to use antinausea medications during pregnancy as women whose fetuses did not have CHD. The difference was statistically significant.

2. There was no difference in the use of tranquilizers between the study group and the control group.

3. Women with CHD fetuses had an average age of 23 years versus 18 years for women whose fetuses did not have CHD. The results were statistically significant.

4. The women with CHD fetuses drank an average of 3.7 cups of coffee per day, whereas women whose fetuses did not have CHD drank an average of 3.5 cups of coffee per day. The differences were statistically significant.

5. Among the other 96 variables studied, the authors found that women with CHD fetuses were twice as likely to have blond hair and to be over 5 ft. 6 in. tall. Both differences were statistically significant using the usual statistical methods.

The authors drew the following conclusions:

1. Antinausea medications cause CHD since they are more often used by women whose fetuses have CHD.
2. Tranquilizers are safe for use in pregnancy since they were not associated with an increased risk of CHD.
3. Since women in their twenties are more likely to have fetuses with CHD, women should be encouraged to have their children before the age of 20.
4. Since coffee drinking increases the risk of CHD, coffee drinking should be eliminated completely during pregnancy, which would largely eliminate the risk of CHD.
5. Despite the fact that no one had hypothesized height and hair color as risk factors for CHD, these were proved to be important predictors of CHD.

CRITIQUE: EXERCISE NO. 1

Study Design

The investigators have not clarified the aims of their study. Are they interested in specific types of CHD? Congenital heart disease consists of a variety of conditions involving valves, septum, and blood vessels. In lumping all conditions under the heading *CHD*, the investigators are assuming that a common etiology exists for all these conditions. In addition, the specific hypotheses being tested are not clarified in this study. The groups chosen consist of a study group who underwent spontaneous abortion and a control group who underwent voluntary induced abortions. These groups can be expected to be different in a variety of ways. It would have been preferable to choose more comparable groups of women, for instance, those who had induced abortions with and without CHD or those who had spontaneous abortions with and without CHD.

With this study design it must be remembered that only CHD that was severe enough to cause early spontaneous abortion is being studied. Although this may provide important information, the factors causing CHD severe enough to abort fetuses may be different from the factors causing CHD in full-term babies.

Assignment

To determine whether a selection bias exists, we ask first if the study group and the control group differ in some respect. Second, we ask if these differences have affected the results. The experiences of women having induced abortions versus women having spontaneous abortions are likely to be different in many ways. It is probable that the women also have different attitudes about their pregnancies, which may affect their use of medications during pregnancy. Such differences between the study group and the control group could affect the results so that selection bias may well be present.

Assessment

The high rate of loss to follow-up of participants suggests the possibility that those who were lost to follow-up had different characteristics. A high rate of loss to follow-up weakens the conclusions that can be drawn from any observed differences. Recall bias on the part of the participants is a possibility, particularly when a traumatic event such as having a child with CHD has occurred and they were asked to frequently recall subjectively remembered events, such as use of medication or coffee consumption. The retrospective reporting of medication use for instance may be influenced by the emotions surrounding the loss of the fetus among those experiencing an unexpected spontaneous abortion. The result may be a closer scrutiny of the memory, leading to a more thorough recall of medication use.

Analysis, Interpretation, And Extrapolation

1. Even if one assumes that the relationship between antinausea medications and CHD was properly derived, it has not been shown that a cause and effect relationship exists. Case-control studies cannot definitively settle the question of which factor is the "cause" and which is the "effect." It is possible that women with CHD fetuses have more nausea and therefore take more antinausea medications. Before a causal relationship is established in the clinical sense of causation (contributory cause), investigators must show that the postulated cause precedes the effect and that altering the cause alters the effect. The authors of this study have made an interpretation that is not necessarily warranted by the data. Performing an adjustment for differences in the frequency of nausea in the study and control groups as part of the analysis would be one method to further evaluate the possible relationship between antinausea medications and CHD while still using a case-control study.

2. The absence of a difference between groups in terms of use of tranquilizers does not necessarily ensure the safety of these drugs. The samples may be too small to fully test the risk of tranquilizers causing CHD. A small increase in risk requires many more study subjects before the investigation has the statistical power to demonstrate a difference between groups with a high level of certainty. Thus, a Type II error may have been committed. Even if there is no risk of tranquilizers causing CHD, this does not ensure that there are not other adverse effects on the fetus that make tranquilizers unsafe for use during pregnancy. The investigators have therefore extrapolated far beyond the data.

3. The difference in age between the two groups of women may be related to both their abortion status and their CHD status. Thus age may be selection bias if women are more likely to undergo induced abortion in their teen-aged years rather than later in life; this relationship alone may explain the differences in age between the groups. Even if the study had shown that the risk of CHD was smaller for teen-aged pregnancies, the medical and social risks of teen-aged pregnancy might outweigh this benefit. The mere presence of a statistically significant difference does not mean that a clinically important conclusion has been reached.

4. The difference between coffee drinkers and noncoffee drinkers is statistically significant, but it is not great. A statistically significant result is one with a low probability of occurring by chance if no true differences exist in the larger populations from which the sample data were drawn. However, it is clinically unlikely that such a small reduction in coffee consumption would have a great effect on the risk of CHD. Statistical significance must be distinguished from clinical importance and from contributory cause. Coffee drinking may have an effect, but with such small differences, one must be careful of concluding too much.

5. By testing 100 variables, it is not surprising that the authors found associations that were statistically significant. When using many variables, one cannot use the usual level of statistical significance to reject the null hypothesis of no association. The usual 5% level assumes one hypothesis is developed prior to the study. Thus, the authors cannot safely conclude that height and hair color are risk factors for CHD.

Alternatively those with a Bayesian approach might say that hair color and height have a low prior probability of being associated with CHD. Thus the fact that one observed an association may well represent a Type I error since the probability of an association after obtaining the results of the study is still relatively low.

EXERCISE NO. 2: COHORT STUDY

In an attempt to study the effects of a well-run cardiac care unit (CCU) on myocardial infarctions (MIs), investigators conducted a concurrent cohort study of the effects of a new CCU.

During the CCU's first year of operation, 100 study group patients with diagnoses of rule-out MI were admitted to the CCU by their attending physicians. One hundred control group patients were admitted by their attending physicians directly to non-CCU ward beds with diagnoses of rule-out MI.

CCU patients were administered lidocaine if cardiac enzymes were positive for MI 24 hours after admission. CCU patients were treated with aggressive interventions to assess and treat occlusions of their coronary arteries. Ward patients were monitored for complications that were then treated.

In comparing the CCU patients with the ward patients, researchers found that the average age for CCU patients was 58 years versus 68 years for the ward patients. One-fourth of the CCU patients developed hypotension versus one-twentieth of the ward patients. Eighty percent of the CCU patients experienced ventricular arrhythmias versus twenty percent of the ward patients. The researchers followed the patients during their hospitalization and for 1 year after hospitalization. They collected the following outcome data:

1. Thirty-six of the CCU patients eventually showed definite electrocardiogram or enzyme evidence of MIs versus thirty of the ward patients.
2. Eight CCU patients died in the hospital versus four ward patients. The differences were not statistically significant.
3. CCU patients remained in the hospital an average of 12 days versus 15 days for ward patients. The differences were statistically significant.
4. Among patients given lidocaine in the CCU, none died.
5. One year after discharge, former CCU patients were able to exercise an average of 20% longer than former ward patients.

The authors then drew the following conclusions:

1. CCU care causes a higher rate of development of MI among patients admitted to the hospital with chest pains.
2. Since the differences in death rates were not statistically significant, CCU patients and ward patients have the same death rate.
3. Since the differences in length of hospitalization were statistically significant, the investigators concluded that they had demonstrated an important cost saving through use of CCU care.
4. Since lidocaine prevented all deaths if used after the definitive diagnosis of MI, use of lidocaine on admission to the CCU would eliminate all mortality due to MIs.
5. Since the CCU patients demonstrated greater exercise tolerance 1 year after discharge, CCU care causes improvement in long-term survival.

CRITIQUE: EXERCISE NO. 2

Study Design

The investigators sought to study the effects of a well-run CCU unit and chose to conduct their study in a new CCU. However, new facilities may not operate at full efficiency during the first year. Thus, the investigators may not have chosen an optimal setting for studying the effects of a well-run CCU. In addition the authors failed to state their specific hypotheses before conducting the study.

Assignment

Selection bias may be present in this study if individuals with a poor prognosis were admitted to the CCU by their attending physicians. This factor could be important if physicians selectively admitted sicker patients with a poor prognosis to the CCU. Then selection bias would be expected to affect the results of the study.

Assessment

The investigators found a much higher rate of arrhythmias among the CCU patients, which may have been the result of the method used for assessing arrhythmias. If CCU patients were monitored continuously whereas those on unmonitored wards were not, it is possible that the intensity of observation of CCU patients uncovered a higher percentage of those arrhthymias that were present.

Analysis

The researchers also found the CCU patients were younger, on the average, than ward patients. This factor may have occurred by chance or it may have resulted from the physicians' desire to provide more intensive care for younger patients. The age of patients is likely to be associated with certain outcomes such as exercise tolerance after MI since younger men on average have great exercise tolerance. Thus, regardless of whether this difference occurred through bias or chance, it resulted in a difference in age. Age differences are a potential confounding variable that should be adjusted for as part of the analysis.

Interpretation And Extrapolation

1. The investigators found that a lower percentage of ward patients eventually showed evidence of a MI and concluded that the higher rate of MIs in CCU patients was caused by CCU care. The first requirement of establishing a cause and effect relationship is to establish that the cause precedes the effect. In this situation, it is likely that the

patients already had experienced or were experiencing MIs when they were admitted to the hospital. Thus, in most cases, the effect (MI) may have preceded the cause (admission to the CCU). There is little evidence to support the interpretation that CCU care causes a higher rate of development of MI.

2. The authors concluded that the death rates should be considered to be the same since no statistically significant difference in death rates occurred. The failure to demonstrate a statistically significant difference does not necessarily imply that no difference exists. When the numbers are few, a very large difference is required to demonstrate statistical significance. The authors have not recognized the possibility of a Type II error. It is likely that more seriously ill patients were admitted to the CCU, so a higher death rate was expected among CCU patients. When the numbers are as few as the number of deaths in this study, it is better simply to state the number of deaths in each group without applying statistical significance tests. In this study a difference did exist; even if the difference is not statistically significant, the observed number of deaths cannot be considered identical.

3. The CCU patients had a shorter length of hospitalization than the ward patients. The results were statistically significant, implying that the differences were not likely to be due to chance. Whether these differences are important from the cost standpoint is another question; the additional costs of CCU care may override the small differences in length of hospitalization. The study itself provides no data to address this issue. This consideration may illustrate the distinction to be made between a statistically significant difference and a clinically important difference.

4. Lidocaine was administered to CCU patients only after a definitive enzyme diagnosis was made and a MI was present at 24 hours. By this time the risk of death from a MI has greatly decreased, especially the arrhythmia risk. It is likely therefore that lidocaine administration has little to do with the fact that no deaths occurred among those given lidocaine. The authors have gone beyond the data in extrapolating their results to all CCU patients and did not recognize that the group of patients on lidocaine was different from patients newly admitted to the CCU.

5. The authors concluded that CCU care improved the prospect of recovery since CCU patients had a better exercise tolerance 1 year later. Insufficient evidence exists to establish a cause and effect relationship. Since CCU patients were younger than ward patients, they could be expected to have a better exercise tolerance. In addition, more CCU patients died. The ability to survive a MI may have produced a group with a higher exercise tolerance. Finally, no evidence is presented that exercise tolerance 1 year after a MI is actually associated with improved long-term survival. The authors should have been more careful about relating a better prognosis to CCU care; in doing so, they extrapolated far beyond the data.

REVIEW EXERCISE: A STUDY OF MEDICAL SCREENING IN A MILITARY POPULATION

During their first year in the military service, 10,000 eighteen-year-old privates were offered the opportunity to participate in a yearly health maintenance examination that included history, physical examination, and multiple laboratory tests. The first year 5,000 participated and 5,000 failed to participate. The 5,000 participants were selected as a study group, and the 5,000 nonparticipants were selected as a control group. The first-year participants were then offered yearly health maintenance examinations during each year of their military service.

On discharge from the military, each of the 5,000 study group members and each of the 5,000 control group members were given an extensive history, physical examination, and laboratory evaluation to determine whether the yearly health maintenance visits had made any difference in the health and life-style of the participants.

The investigators obtained the following information:

1. On the basis of their reported consumption, participants had half the rate of alcoholism as nonparticipants.
2. Participants had twice as many diagnoses made on them during military service as nonparticipants.
3. Participants had advanced an average of twice as many ranks as nonparticipants.
4. No statistically significant differences occurred between the groups in the rate of MI.
5. No differences were found between the groups in the rate of development of testicular cancer or Hodgkin's disease, the two most common cancers in young men.

The authors then drew the following conclusions:

1. Yearly screening can reduce the rate of alcoholism in the entire military by one-half.

2. Since participants had twice the number of diagnoses made on them, their diseases were being diagnosed at an earlier stage in the disease process, at a point where therapy is more beneficial.
3. Since participants had twice the military advancement of nonparticipants, the screening program must have contributed to the quality of their work.
4. Since no difference occurred between the groups in the rate of MI, screening and intervention for coronary risk factors should not be included in a future health maintenance screening program.
5. Since testicular cancer and Hodgkin's disease occurred with equal frequency in both groups, future health maintenance examinations should not include efforts to diagnose these conditions.

CRITIQUE: REVIEW EXERCISE

Study Design

The investigators have stated only a general goal of studying the value of the annual health maintenance examination. They do not target the population to which they wish to apply their results. They do not state specific hypotheses or clearly identify their specific study questions.

If the investigators' goal was to study the effects of an annual health maintenance examination, they have not accomplished this goal since no evidence exists that first-year participants actually took part in subsequent examinations.

Furthermore the authors' choice of study participants may not have been appropriate for the study question. The study selected young persons who already had been screened for chronic illness by virtue of passing the entry physical for military service. Being a young and healthy group, they may not have been an appropriate population for testing the usefulness of health maintenance for older or higher-risk populations such as an older military population in which the frequency of pathologic conditions would be expected to be much higher.

Assignment

Individuals in this study were self-selected; that is, they decided whether or not to participate. The participants therefore can be considered volunteers. The researchers presented no evidence to indicate that those who elected to participate differed in any way from those that elected not to participate. It is likely that participants had health habits and health risks that were different from those of the nonpartic-ipants. These differences may well have contributed to the differences in the outcome. Since no baseline evaluation is available on the control group, it is not known if or how they differed from the study group. Thus, one does not know if the study group and the control group were comparable.

The individuals in both the study and control groups were self-assigned on the basis of their participation in the first year of the health maintenance examinations. Since the examinations were con-ducted on a yearly basis, those who initially participated may not have continued to participate. Thus, the study or control group status of the individuals involved may not have validly reflected their actual participation in the screening.

Assessment

Assessment of outcome was conducted only on those who were dis-charged from the military. Those who remained in the military would not have been included. Individuals who had died during military service would not have been included in those assessed at discharge. The individuals who had died may have been the most important in terms of assessing the potential benefits gained by screening.

Individuals participating in multiple health maintenance examina-tions were under much more intensive observation than the nonpar-ticipants. The unequal intensity of observation may have resulted in a greater number of diagnoses being made for them during their mili-tary service. Nonparticipants may have had the same number of con-ditions, but not all of them resulted in a recorded diagnosis.

Analysis, Interpretation, And Extrapolation

1. Participants had a lower rate of alcoholism than nonparticipants, perhaps as a result of differences between the groups prior to entry into the study. If heavy drinkers were less likely to participate in the health screening, then the screening would only appear to have altered the frequency of alcoholism. Comparative baseline data and adjustment for the differences were lacking in the analysis. In ad-dition, the validity of the method used for assessment of alcohol consumption is questionable. Since no uniform criteria existed for diagnosis, differences in recall and reporting were possible. Even if none of these potential errors existed, there is no evidence in the study that the screening itself was the causative factor in producing a lower rate of alcoholism. Extrapolating to the military in general went well beyond the range of the data.

2. If a higher level of motivation is associated both with the participation in the study and advancement in the military, then motivation would be a confounding variable, one related to both the participation status and the outcome. Without controlling for this potentially confounding variable, no conclusion can be reached about the relationship between participation status and advancement.

3. Many of those with MI may have died, and thus were excluded from the assessment. In addition, one would expect a very low rate of MI in a young population. Even with the great numbers included in this study, the sample may not have been big enough to demonstrate statistically significant differences for real but small differences between the groups. If one assumes that alterations in the risk factors that contribute to MI also alter the prognosis, no indication exists here that those who participated had either more recognized risk factors or more risk factors altered. Even if they had more altered risk factors, the effects of these alterations may not become apparent until years after the participants have left the military. Therefore, this study was incapable of answering the question of whether screening for risk factors for coronary artery disease alters prognosis.

4. The absence of differences in the rate of development of testicular cancer and Hodgkin's disease cannot be assessed on the basis of those discharged alive. Even if the rates of development of the disease were identical, they say little about the success or failure of the screening program. A cancer screening program aims to pick up disease at an early stage; it does not aim to prevent disease. Thus the rate of development of cancer cannot be used to evaluate the success or failure of a screening program. Therefore, one would expect nearly identical rates of development of Hodgkin's and testicular carcinoma. The stage of illness at diagnosis and the prognosis for those who developed either of the conditions would be more appropriate measures for assessing the success of the screening program. No such data are presented here, and thus, no interpretation can be made.

Having critiqued these flaw-catching exercises, the reader may feel discouraged, but, of course, most medical research studies have far fewer errors than the hypothetical exercises presented here. However, it may help the reader to remember that a certain number of errors are unavoidable, and that detecting errors is not the same as invalidating research.

The practice of clinical medicine requires that clinicians act on probabilities; therefore, a critical reading of the medical literature helps the clinician to more accurately define these probabilities. The art of reading the medical literature is the ability to draw useful conclusions from uncertain data. Learning to detect errors not only helps the clinician to recognize the limitations of a particular study, but also helps to temper the tendency to automatically put into practice the newest research results.

CHAPTER 11

Interventional Studies: Controlled Clinical Trials

Controlled clinical trials have increasingly become the gold standard by which we judge the benefits of therapy. The Federal Drug Administration (FDA) requires them for drug approval, the National Institutes of Health (NIH) rewards them by funding, the journals encourage them by publication, and increasingly, clinicians read them for certainty. When feasible and ethical, controlled clinical trials have become a standard part of clinical research. Thus it is critically important to appreciate what controlled clinical trials can tell us, what can go wrong, and what questions they cannot address. To accomplish this we will use the uniform framework for clinical studies and discuss the elements of study design, assignment, assessment, analysis, interpretation, and extrapolation with respect to controlled clinical trials.

UNIFORM FRAMEWORK FOR CLINICAL TRIALS

Study Design

Controlled clinical trials are able to demonstrate all three criteria of contributory cause. When applied to a treatment, the term *efficacy* is used instead of *contributory cause*.* By *efficacy* we mean that the therapy produces a reduction in the probability or risk of experiencing the

---

* A technique that removes a contributory cause by definition has efficacy. However, removing as indirect contributory cause may still have efficacy even after the state of knowledge has allowed us to define a more direct contributory cause.

adverse outcome in the study group being investigated. *Efficacy*, however, needs to be distinguished from *effectiveness*. *Effectiveness* implies that the therapy works under usual conditions of clinical practice as opposed to the conditions of an investigation. Our goal usually is to use controlled clinical trials to determine if the therapy works when given according to a defined dosage schedule, by a defined route of administration, to a defined type of patient.*

Controlled clinical trials are not suited to the initial investigation of a new treatment. When used as part of the drug approval process, controlled clinical trials are frequently referred to as *Phase III trials*. As defined by the FDA, *Phase I* trials refer to the initial efforts to administer the treatment to human beings. They aim to establish a dosage regimen and to evaluate the potential toxicities. They provide only a preliminary look at the potential efficacy of the therapy. *Phase II trials* aim to establish the indications and regimen for administration of the new therapy and to determine whether the new therapy warrants further study. Phase II studies are usually small-scale controlled or uncontrolled trials that aim to establish whether a full-scale controlled clinical trial should be conducted.

Ideally a controlled clinical or Phase III trial should be performed after the indications and the regimen are agreed on but before the therapy has been widely integrated into clinical care. For new drugs that do not have market approval, this is relatively automatic. However, for many procedures and drugs that have been previously marketed, the treatment may have been widely used before controlled clinical trials can be implemented. This is a problem since once the treatment has been widely used, physicians and often patients have developed firm ideas about the value of the therapy. If physicians or patients already have firm ideas about the value of the therapy, they may not feel that it is ethical to enter into an experimental trial or to continue participation if they discover that the patient had been assigned to the control group.

Having decided that the time is right for a controlled clinical trial, the next study design question is, is it feasible? To understand what is feasible one must define the question in a controlled clinical trial.

Most controlled clinical trials aim to determine whether the new or experimental therapy results in a better outcome than placebo or standard therapy. To determine whether a trial is feasible, investigators need to estimate the necessary sample size. They need to estimate how many patients are required to have a reasonable chance of demon-

---

* It is possible to perform a controlled clinical trial to assess the effectiveness of therapy by using a representative sample of the types of patients to be treated with the therapy and the usual methods that will be used clinically.

strating a statistically significant difference between the new therapy and the placebo or standard therapy.

The required sample size is dependent on the following factors:*

1. The size of the Type I error that the investigators will tolerate. This is the probability of demonstrating a statistically significant difference in samples when no true difference exists between treatments in the large populations. The alpha level for the Type I error is usually set at 5%.

2. The size of the Type II error that the investigators will tolerate. This is the probability of failing to demonstrate a statistically significant difference in samples when a true difference of a selected magnitude actually exists between treatments. Most investigators aim for no more than a 20% Type II error. A 20% Type II error is also referred to as an 80% statistical power. The 80% power implies 80% probability of being able to demonstrate a statistically significant difference if a true difference exists.

3. The percentage of individuals in the control group who are expected to experience the adverse outcome (death or development of disease) under study. Often this can be estimated from previous studies.

4. The improvement in outcome among those in the study group that one seeks to demonstrate as statistically significant. Despite the desire to demonstrate statistical significance for even small real changes, the investigators need to decide the size of a difference that would be considered clinically important. The smaller this difference between study group and control group therapy that one expects to observe, the larger the sample size required.

Let us take a look at the way these factors affect the required sample size. Table 11-1 provides general guidelines for sample size for different levels of these factors.

Table 11-1 assumes one study group and one control group of equal size. It also assumes that one is interested in the study results whether they are in the direction of the study treatment or in the opposite direction. Statisticians refer to statistical significance tests that consider data favoring deviation from the null hypothesis in either direction as two-tailed tests. Table 11-1 also assumes a Type I error of 5%.

---

* This is all the information that is required for an either/or variable. When calculating sample size for variables with multiple possible outcomes, one must also estimate the standard deviation of the variable.

TABLE 11-1. SAMPLE SIZE REQUIREMENT FOR CONTROLLED CLINICAL TRIALS

			Probability of Adverse Outcome in the Study Group			
			1%	5%	10%	20%
		TYPE II ERROR				
	2%	10%	3,696	851	207	72
		20%	2,511	652	161	56
		50%	1,327	351	90	38
Probability of Adverse Outcome in the Control Group	10%	10%	154	619		285
		20%	120	473		218
		50%	69	251		117
	20%	10%	62	112	285	
		20%	49	87	218	
		50%	29	49	117	
	40%	10%	25	33	48	117
		20%	20	26	37	90
		50%	12	16	22	49
	60%	10%	13	16	20	34
		20%	11	13	16	27
		50%	7	8	10	16

Let us take a look at the meaning of these numbers for different types of studies. Imagine that we wish to conduct a controlled clinical trial on a treatment designed to reduce the 1-year death rate of adenocarcinoma of the ovary. Let us assume that the 1-year death rate using standard therapy is 40%. In this study we hope to be able to reduce the 1-year death rate to 20% using a new treatment. We believe, however, that the treatment could possibly increase the death rate. If we are willing to tolerate a 20% probability of failing to obtain statistically significant results, even if a true difference of this magnitude exists in the larger populations, how many patients are required in the study and the control groups?

To answer this question we can use Table 11-1 as follows: Locate the 20% probability of an adverse outcome in the study group on the horizontal axis. Next locate the 40% probability of an adverse outcome in the control group on the vertical axis. These intersect in the box that contains 117, 90, and 49. The correct one is the one that lines up with the 20% Type II error. The answer is 90. Thus 90 women with advance adenocarcinoma in the study group and 90 control group women are needed to have a 20% probability of failing to demonstrate statistical significance if the true 1-year death rate is actually 40% using the standard treatment and 20% using the new therapy.

A sample size of 100 is a commonly used sample size for controlled clinical trials. It is an approximate estimate of the number of individuals needed in each group when the probability of an adverse outcome is substantial and the investigators hope to be able to reduce it in half with the new treatment while keeping the size of the Type II error less than 20%.

Now let us contrast this situation with one in which the probability of an adverse outcome is much lower even without intervention.

An investigator wishes to study the effect of a new treatment on the risk of neonatal sepsis secondary to delayed presentation of premature rupture of the membranes. We will assume that the risk of neonatal sepsis using standard treatment is 10%, and the study group therapy aims to reduce the risk of neonatal sepsis to 5% though it is possible that the new therapy will increase the death rate. The investigator is willing to tolerate a 10% probability of failing to demonstrate a statistically significant difference.

Using the chart as before, we located 619, 473, and 251. Thus we see that 619 individuals are necessary for the study group and 619 individuals are necessary for the control group to ensure a 10% probability of making a Type II error. If we were willing to tolerate a 20% probability of failing to demonstrate a statistically significant difference, if a difference actually exists in the larger populations, 473 individuals would be required in each group. Five hundred individuals in each group is usually a large number for a controlled clinical trial. Yet this is the approximate size that is required if we wish to be able to demonstrate statistical significance when the true difference between adverse outcomes in the larger population is only 10% versus 5%. The neonatal sepsis example is typical of the problems we study in clinical practice. It demonstrates why large sample sizes are required in most controlled clinical trials before it is feasible to demonstrate statistical significance. Thus, it is not usually feasible to submit small improvements in therapy to the test of a controlled clinical trial.

Let us go one step further and see what happens to the required sample size when a controlled clinical trial is performed on a preventive intervention in which the adverse outcome is uncommon even in the absence of prevention.

Imagine that a new drug to prevent adverse outcomes of pregnancy in women who are hypertensive prior to pregnancy aims to reduce the risk of adverse pregnancy outcomes from 2% to 1% though it is possible that the new therapy will increase the death rate. The investigators are willing to tolerate a 20% probability of failing to demonstrate a statistically significant difference.

From Table 11-1 we can see that 2,511 individuals are required in each group. These enormous numbers point out the difficulty in performing controlled clinical trials when one wishes to apply preventive therapy, especially when the risk of adverse outcomes is already quite low.

Even when a controlled clinical trial is feasible, it may not be ethical to perform. Controlled clinical trials are not considered ethical if they require individuals to submit to substantial risks without a realistic expectation of a substantial benefit. For instance, a trial of unopposed high-dose estrogen therapy today would not be permitted by an institutional review board whose approval is required before individuals are allowed to volunteer for a study. Thus despite the advantages of clinical trials in defining the efficacy of a therapy, a controlled clinical trial may not always be feasible or ethical.

Assignment

Individuals included in a randomized controlled trial are not usually selected at random from a larger population. Usually they are volunteers who meet a series of entry and exclusion criteria set up by the investigators.

Volunteers for an investigation must provide informed consent that must include an explanation of the known risks and available alternatives. Volunteers have the right to withdraw from the study at any time for any reason; however, they do not have a right to know their treatment group assignment while in the study and are not usually eligible to receive compensation through the investigation for adverse side effects of therapy.

The randomization of patients to study and control groups is the hallmark of controlled clinical trials. Randomization implies that any one individual has a predetermined probability of being assigned to each particular study and control group. This may mean an equal probability of being assigned to one study and one control group or different probabilities of being assigned to each of several study and control groups.

Randomization is a powerful tool for eliminating selection bias in the assignment of individuals to study and control groups. In large studies it helps reduce the possibility that the effects of treatment are due to the type of individuals receiving the study and control therapy. It is important to distinguish between randomization, which is an essential part of a controlled clinical trial, and random selection, which is not usually a part of a controlled clinical trial. Random selection as opposed to randomization implies that the individuals who are selected for a study are selected by chance from a larger group or population. Thus random selection is a method aimed at obtaining a representative sample (i.e., one that reflects the characteristics of a larger group).

Randomization on the other hand says nothing about the characteristics of a large population from which the individuals in the investigation are obtained. It refers to the mechanism by which individuals are assigned to study and control groups once they become eligible for and volunteer for the study. The following hypothetical study illustrates the difference between random selection and randomization.

An investigator wishes to assess the benefit of a new drug known as "Surf-ez." Surf-ez is designed to help improve surfing ability. To assess the value of Surf-ez the investigator performs a randomized controlled clinical trial among a group of volunteer championship surfers in Hawaii. After randomization of half the group to Surf-ez and half the group to a placebo, the surfing ability of all surfers is measured using a standard scoring system. The scorers do not know whether the surfers used Surf-ez or placebo. Those taking Surf-ez have a statistically significant and substantial improvement compared to the placebo group. Based on the results of the study, the authors recommend Surf-ez as a learning aid for all surfers.

By using randomization, this controlled clinical trial has demonstrated the efficacy of Surf-ez among these championship surfers. However, since its study and control groups were hardly a random sample of surfers, we need to be very careful in drawing conclusions about the effects of Surf-ez as a learning aid for all surfers.*

Randomization does not eliminate the possibility that study and control groups will differ according to factors that affect prognosis (confounding variables). Known prognostic factors must still be measured and will often be found to be different in study and control groups due to chance alone, especially in small studies. If substantial differences between groups exist, these need to be taken into account through an adjustment process as part of the analysis.† Many characteristics affecting prognosis, however, are not known. In larger studies randomization tends to balance the multitude of characteristics that could possibly be related to outcome, even those that are unknown to the investigator. Without randomization the investigator would need to take into account all known and potential differences

---

* Care must be taken even in extrapolating to championship surfers since we have not randomly sampled all championship surfers. This limitation occurs in most controlled clinical trials, which select their patients from a particular hospital or clinical site.

† Many biostatisticians would recommend use of a multivariable analysis technique such as regression analysis even when no substantial difference exists between groups. Use of multivariable analyses then permits adjustment for interaction. Interaction occurs for instance when both groups contain an identical age and sex distribution but one group contains predominantly young females and the other contains predominantly young males. Multivariable analysis then allows one to separate out the interacting effects of age and sex.

between groups. Since it is difficult if not impossible to consider everything, randomization helps balance the groups, especially for large studies.

Assessment

Blinding of study subjects and investigators is often considered an important characteristic in the design of controlled clinical trials to prevent errors in assessment of outcome. *Single blinding* implies that the patient is unaware of which therapy is being received; *double blinding* implies that neither the patient nor the investigator is aware of the group assignment.

Errors in assessing the outcome or end point of a controlled clinical trial may occur when the patient or the individual making the assessment is aware of which treatment is being administered. This is especially likely when the outcome or end point being measured is subjective or may be influenced by knowledge of the treatment group as illustrated in the following hypothetical study:

A randomized controlled clinical trial of a new breast cancer surgery compared the degree of arm edema and strength in the new procedure versus the traditional procedure. The patients were aware of which procedure they underwent. Arm edema and arm strength were the end points assessed by the patients and surgeons. The study found that those receiving the new procedure had less arm edema and more arm strength than those undergoing the traditional mastectomy.

In this study the fact that the patients and the surgeons who performed the procedure and assessed the outcome all knew which patient received which procedure may have affected the objectivity of the way strength and edema were measured and reported. This effect may have been minimized but not totally eliminated if individuals who were not aware which patient received which therapy assessed arm strength and edema using a standardized quantitative scoring system. This system of blind assessment and objective scoring would minimize the impact of the fact that the patients and surgeons knew which surgery was obtained. However, it is still possible that patients receiving the new procedure worked harder to increase their strength and reduce their edema. This could occur for instance if the surgeon performing the new surgery stressed postoperative exercises more forcefully among those receiving the new therapy.

In practice, blinding is often impractical or unsuccessful. Surgical therapy cannot easily be blinded. The taste or side effects of medications are often a giveaway to the patient, the physician, or both. The need to titrate a dose to achieve a desired effect often makes it more difficult to blind the physician and in some cases the patient. Strict adherence to blinding helps ensure the objectivity of the assessment process. It helps remove the possibility that differences in compliance, follow-through, and assessment of outcome will be affected by awareness of the treatment being received.

Even when objective assessment, excellent compliance, and complete follow-up can be ensured, blinding is still desirable since it helps control for the placebo effect. The placebo effect is a powerful biological process that can bring about a wide variety of objective as well as subjective biological effects. The placebo effect extends far beyond pain control. A substantial percentage of patients who believe they are receiving effective therapy obtain objective therapeutic benefits. When effective blinding is not a part of a controlled clinical trial, it leaves open the possibility that the observed benefit in the study subject is actually the result of the placebo therapy.

Thus when blinding is not feasible, doubt about the accuracy of the outcome measures will usually remain. This uncertainty can be reduced but not eliminated by use of objective measures of end points, careful monitoring of compliance, and complete follow-up of patients.

Valid assessment of outcome requires measures of outcome that are appropriate, precise, complete, and unaffected by the process of observation. The requirements are as important in a controlled clinical trial as in a case-control and cohort study as we discussed in Chapter 4.

In an ideal controlled clinical trial, all individuals would be treated according to the study protocol and followed forward in time. Their outcome would be assessed from their time of entry right up to the end of the study. In reality, assessment is rarely so perfect or complete. Patients often receive treatment that deviates from the predefined protocol. Investigators often label these individuals as *protocol deviants.* In addition some patients are usually lost to follow-up before the end of the study.

Biases can arise in controlled clinical trials from these protocol deviants and from patients lost to follow-up. Let us see how this might occur by looking at the following hypothetical study:

In a controlled clinical trial of renal dialysis, 100 patients were randomized to daily dialysis and 100 patients to weekly intensive dialysis. During the course of the study, 2 patients receiving daily dialysis deviated from the protocol and received a kidney transplant, and 20 patients from the weekly dialysis treatment deviated from the protocol and received transplantation. The investigators eliminated from the study those who went on to transplantation, feeling that their inclusion would unfairly affect the study results.

It is possible that many of these who underwent transplantation were doing poorly with their dialysis treatment. If this is the case, exclusion of those who deviated from the protocol would bias the results of the study in favor of the weekly dialysis group. This would occur if those remaining in the weekly dialysis group included mainly those who were doing well.

Because of the potential bias, it is generally recommended that deviants from the study protocol remain in the investigation and be subsequently analyzed as if they had remained in the group to which they were originally randomized. This is known as *analysis according to the intention to treat.* By retaining the protocol deviants, the study question, however, is changed slightly. The study now asks whether a policy of implementing the new treatment as much as possible is superior to a policy of implementing the standard therapy as much as possible. This change may actually help make the investigation more applicable to the real clinical questions, or in other words the effectiveness of the therapy as actually used in clinical practice.

Deviations from the protocol are relatively common in controlled clinical trials since it is considered unethical to prevent deviations when the attending physician feels that continued adherence is contraindicated by the patient's condition or when the patient no longer wishes to follow the recommended protocol. Thus in evaluating a controlled clinical trial, the reader should understand the degree of protocol adherence and determine how the investigators handled the data on those who deviated from the protocol.

A similar problem can occur when individuals are lost to follow-up prior to the completion of a study. Even moderate loss to follow-up can be disastrous for a study if those lost move to Arizona because of failing health, drop out because of drug toxicity, or fail to return due to the burdens of compliance with one of the treatment protocols.

Well-conducted studies make elaborate precautions to minimize the loss to follow-up. In some cases follow-up may be completed by a telephone or mail questionnaire. A search of death records should be made for those who cannot be located. When loss to follow-up occurs despite these precautions, it is important to determine, as much as possible, the initial characteristics of patients subsequently lost to follow-up. This is done in an attempt to determine whether those lost are likely to be different from those who remain. If those lost to follow-up have an especially poor prognosis, little may be gained by analyzing the data from those who remain as suggested by the following hypothetical study:

In a study of the effects of a new alcohol treatment program, 100 patients were randomized to a new alcohol treatment program, and 100 patients were randomized to conventional treatment. The investigators visited the homes of all patients at 9 o'clock on a Saturday night and drew blood from all available patients in order to measure alcohol levels. Of the new treatment group, 30 patients were at home, and one-third of these had alcohol in their blood. Among the conventionally treated patients, 40 were at home, and one-half of these had alcohol in their blood.

Whenever more than a small loss to follow-up or a disproportionate loss in one group occurs, it is important to ask what happened to those that were lost to follow-up. In this study, if those lost to follow-up were out drinking, the results based on those at home would be especially misleading.

One method for dealing with loss to follow-up is to assume the worst for those lost to follow-up. For instance one would assume that all those not at home were out drinking. It is then possible to redo the analysis and compare the outcome in the study and control groups. When the loss to follow-up is great, this procedure will usually leave one without a substantial or statistically significant difference between the study and control groups. However, for smaller loss to follow-up, a statistically significant difference may remain. When statistically significant differences between groups remain after assuming the worst case for those lost to follow-up, then the reader can be quite confident that loss to follow-up does not explain the observed differences.

Analysis

Two basic analysis questions face the investigator in a controlled clinical trial: when to analyze the data and how to analyze the data.

When To Analyze Data

The seemingly simple question of when to analyze has provoked considerable methodologic and ethical controversy. The more times one analyzes, the more likely one is to find a point when the P value reaches the 0.05 level of statistical significance.

When to analyze is an ethical problem since one would like to establish that a true difference exists at the earliest possible moment. This is desirable in order to avoid subjecting patients to less effective therapy. In addition, it is desirable that other patients receive an effective therapy at the earliest possible time.

A series of "sequential" methods have been developed to attempt to deal with these problems. These methods have been most successfully applied in studies of acute disease in which the outcome is known in a very short period of time. Most studies, however, rely on the technique of performing analyses at predetermined times. Thus, it is important to understand when and how often to analyze. Ideally, times are determined prior to initiating the study, corresponding to periods when a therapeutic effect would be expected. Thus for antibiotic therapy of an acute disease, the end point may be assessed on a daily basis. For a study of cancer mortality, the end point may be measured only on a yearly basis. When multiple points of analysis are planned, statistical techniques are available to take into account the multiple analyses when calculating the P value.

How To Analyze Data

Life tables are the most commonly used method of analysis designed for controlled clinical trials. Life tables are a means of displaying how often and when the adverse outcomes occur.

In this discussion the adverse effect under study will be referred to as death. However, life tables can be used for other effects such as permanent loss of vision or the occurrence of desired effects such as pregnancy after infertility therapy.

Let us begin by discussing why life tables are often necessary in controlled clinical trials. We will then discuss the assumptions underlying their use and demonstrate how they should be interpreted.

In most controlled clinical trials, individuals are entered into the study and randomized over a period of time, as they present for care. In addition, because of late entry, death, or loss to follow-up, individuals are actually followed for various periods of time after entry. Therefore, many of the patients included in a study are not followed for the full duration of the study.

If all individuals are followed for the same period of time the probability of death can be calculated simply as those dead at the end of the study divided by those initially enrolled in the study. All individuals, however, are not usually followed for the same period of time. Thus life tables provide a method for using the data from those individuals who have been included in a study for only a portion of the possible study duration.* Thus life tables allow the investigator to use all the data that they have so painstakingly collected.

The life-table method is built on the important assumption that those who were in the investigation for shorter time periods would have had the same subsequent experience as those who were actually followed for longer periods

---

* Variations of this type of cohort life table are known as a Kaplan-Meier or Cutter-Ederer life table. Cohort life tables must be distinguished from cross-sectional life tables which are used to estimate life expectancy.

of time. In other words, the "short-termers" would have the same results as the "long-termers" if they were actually followed long-term.

This critical assumption may not hold true if the short-termers are individuals with a better or worse prognosis than the long-termers. This can occur if the entry requirements for the investigation are relaxed during the course of a study. Let us see how this might occur by looking at the next hypothetical study.

A new hormonal treatment designed to treat infertility secondary to severe endometriosis was compared to standard therapy using a controlled clinical trial. After initial difficulty recruiting patients and initial failures to get pregnant among the study patients, one woman in the study group became pregnant. News of her delivery became front-page news. Subsequent patients recruited for the study are found to have much less severe endometriosis, but the investigators willingly accepted those patients and combined their data with data from their original group of patients.

As this study demonstrates, entry criteria may be relaxed if only severely ill patients are entered into an investigation at the beginning. As the therapy becomes better known in the community, at a particular institution, or in the literature, a tendency may occur for the physicians to refer, or patients to self-refer, the less severely ill. In this case, the short-termers are likely to be less severely ill and thus have better outcomes than the long-termers. This problem can be minimized if the investigators clearly define and carefully adhere to a protocol that defines the type of patients who are eligible for the study based on characteristics related to prognosis. Alternatively, they can recognize the problem and statistically adjust their data to take into account the patients' severity of disease at the time of the entry into the study.

Loss to follow-up may also result in differences between the short-termers and the long-termers. This is likely to occur if loss to follow-up occurs preferentially among those who are not doing well or who have adverse reactions to treatment. We have already discussed the importance of loss to follow-up and stressed the need to assess whether those lost are similar to those who remain.

Life-table data are usually presented as a survival plot. This is a graph with the vertical axis showing the percentage survival going from 100% at the top to 0% at the bottom. Thus at the beginning of the investigation, both study and control groups start at the 100% mark at the top of the vertical axis.* The horizontal axis depicts the time of follow-up. Time is counted for each individual beginning with their

---

* Alternatively a graphic presentation of life tables may display the percentage who experience the adverse effect and start at the 0% point on the bottom of the vertical axis.

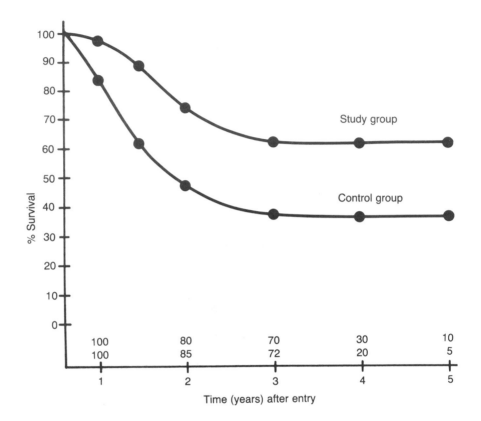

FIGURE 11-1 *A typical study and control group life table demonstrating plateau effect, which typically occurs at the right end of life table plots.*

entry into the study. Thus time zero is not the time in which the investigation began. Survival plots should also include the number of individuals who have been followed for each time interval. Ideally these should be presented separately for the study and the control group. Thus a typical life table comparing the 5-year data on a study and control group might look like Figure 11-1. When life-table data are quoted to estimate the percentage death or survival at, for instance, 5 years, this is known as the *actuarial* 5-year survival. The numbers on the bottom indicate the number of individuals being followed in the study and the control groups up to a particular time after their entry into the study.

Life tables are often tested for statistical significance by use of the log rank or Mantel-Haenszel statistical significance tests. The null hypothesis of these tests states that no difference exists between the overall life tables for the study and control groups. These tests compare the observed and expected events if the null hypothesis of no difference between the study and control group were true. In performing these statistical significance tests, one combines data from each interval in time, taking into account or weighting for the number of individuals being followed during that time interval. Thus these tests combine data from different time intervals to produce an overall statistical significance test. The combination of data from multiple intervals means that the statistical significance test asks this question: If no true difference exists between the overall effects of the study and control group treatments, what is the probability of obtaining the observed or more extreme results? In other words if a statistically significant improvement in a study group has been demonstrated based on life-table curves, it is then very likely that a similar group of individuals receiving the study group therapy will experience at least some improvement compared to the control group therapy.

Interpretation

Data from life tables are prone to a number of misinterpretations as previously discussed. When displaying life-table data, it is important to display the number of individuals being followed at each interval of time in the study and in the control groups. Usually, the number of individuals being followed for the complete duration of a study is few. For instance in Figure 11-1 only 10 individuals are followed for 5 years in the study group and only 5 individuals are followed in the control group. This is not surprising since it often requires some time to start up a study, and these individuals followed for the longest time were recruited during the first year of the study.

A 5-year actuarial survival may be calculated even when only one patient has been followed for 5 years. Thus, one must be very careful not to place too great a reliance on the specific 1-year, 5-year, or any other final probability of survival observed unless the number of individuals actually followed for the full length of the study is great.

In interpreting controlled clinical trial results, it is important to look at the degree of confidence one can place in the survival estimates. Failure to recognize this uncertainty can result in the following type of misinterpretation:

A clinician looking at the life-table curves in Figure 11-1 concluded that 5-year survival with the study treatment is 60% versus 35% with the control group. After extensive use of the same treatment on similar patients, he was surprised that the study treatment actually produced a 55% survival versus only a 50% survival among control group patients.

If the clinician had recognized that life-table curves do not reliably predict exact 5-year survival, he would not have been surprised about his subsequent experience.

Knowledge of the procedures and assumptions underlying life tables also helps in understanding their interpretation. Many survival plots have a flat or plateau phase for long time periods at the right-hand end of the plot. These may be misinterpreted as indicating a cure once an individual reaches the flat or plateau area of the life-table curve. Actually this plateau phase usually results because few individuals are followed for the entire duration of the study. Among those few individuals followed for longer time periods, the deaths are likely to be fewer in number and more widely spaced. Since the survival curve only declines with a death, a plateau is likely when fewer deaths are possible. Thus, in interpreting a life table it is important to understand the *plateau effect*. We should not interpret the plateau as demonstrating a cure unless great numbers of patients have been followed for long periods of time.

In addition to the danger of placing too great a reliance on 5-year actuarial survival derived from a life table and the danger of misinterpreting the plateau, it is important to fully appreciate the interpretation of a statistically significant difference between survival curves. In the study depicted in Figure 11-1, a statistically significant difference occurred in outcome between the study and control groups based on the 5-year actuarial follow-up. The study was subsequently extended for one more year resulting in the life-table curves depicted in Figure 11-2 in which the 6-year actuarial survival was identical in the study and control groups. Based on the 6-year actuarial data, the authors stated that the 5-year actuarial study was mistaken in drawing the conclusion that the study therapy prolonged survival.

Remember that a statistically significant difference in survival curves implies that patients receiving one treatment do better than patients receiving another treatment when taking into account each group's entire experience. Patients in one group may do better only early in the course, midway through, or only at the end. Patients who received the better overall treatment may actually do worse early in the treatment because of surgical complications or at a later point in time as secondary complications develop for those who survive.

Thus when conducting a study, it is important to know enough about the natural history of a disease and the life expectancy of the individuals in the investigation to chose a meaningful time period for follow-up. If the time period is too short, for instance before the

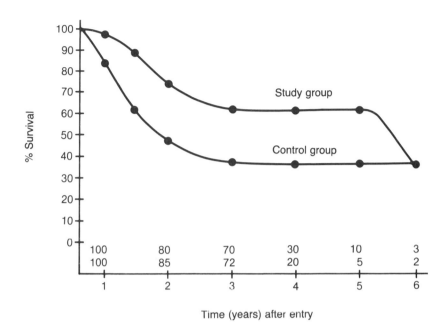

FIGURE 11-2   *Life table plots may meet after extended periods of follow-up. The difference between the overall plots may still be statistically significant.*

therapy is completed, or can be expected to have a biologic effect, differences in outcomes are unlikely.

Similarly follow-up periods that are too long may not allow the study to demonstrate statistically significant differences if the risks of competing diseases overwhelm the shorter-term benefits. For instance a study that assesses the 20-year outcome among 65-year-olds given a treatment for coronary artery disease might show little difference at 20 years even if differences occur at 5 and 10 years.

Use of a survival curve and use of statistical significance testing provide information on the success of the study and control groups' treatment. The interpretation of this effect, however, is aided if we consider whether the groups differ according to a factor or factors known to affect prognosis. These factors are called *confounding variables* if they differ between study and control groups and are related to the probability of an adverse outcome.

One method of dealing with differences in prognostic factors between the groups is to separate or stratify patients according to their prognosis at the beginning of a study and then randomize individuals from each prognostic category or strata to study and control groups. This type of blocked or stratified randomization is a form of group matching that is often used in controlled clinical trials. Alternatively it is also possible to take these differences into account at the end of the study using an *adjustment procedure.*

Adjustment for prognostic factors requires that the information on prognostic or risk factors be collected at the beginning of the study. If differences between the groups are substantial, and these factors are strong prognosticators of outcome, one can take the differences into account using an adjustment procedure. When using life-table methods, it is possible to calculate an adjusted statistical significance test that adds up the observed and expected outcome in each of the different strata of prognosis as well as in the different intervals of time.* The graphic display of the life-table data itself is often not adjusted, though it can be. The statistical significance test should take into account adjustment for confounding variables. Thus when interpreting a statistical significance test performed on a life table, it is important to know whether the procedure has been adjusted for important confounding variables.

We have repeatedly emphasized the distinction between a statistically significant association and a cause and effect relationship. A cause and effect relationship requires the existence of an association. Second, it requires a demonstration that the cause precedes the effect. Third, it requires that altering the cause alters the effect. One of the intellectually satisfying aspects of controlled clinical trials is that they incorporate methods for helping establish all three criteria for contributory cause and thus establish the efficacy of a therapy:

1. Using randomization and adjustment techniques, the investigators are able to produce study and control groups that are comparable except for the effects of the treatment being given. Thus when great and statistically significant differences in outcome occur, the investigator can usually conclude that these differences are associated with the treatment itself.

2. By randomizing individuals to study and control groups at the beginning of the study, the investigator can provide strong evidence that the treatment precedes the effect and is therefore a prior association, fulfilling criterion No. 2 of contributory cause.

3. By providing a treatment that alters the disease process and comparing the treatment and control groups' outcomes, the investigators can provide evidence that the treatment itself (the cause) is actually

---

* This method can be used for nominal or ordinal confounding variables. Methods used to adjust for continuous confounding variables are discussed in Chapter 29.

altering the outcome (the effect), thus fulfilling the third and final criterion for contributory cause.

Controlled clinical trials therefore can help establish the existence of an association between treatment and outcome, can establish the existence of a prior association, and can demonstrate that altering the treatment alters the outcome. These are the three criteria necessary for establishing that the new treatment is the cause of the improved outcome. These criteria establish the efficacy of treatment. It is always possible, however, that unrecognized effects other than the intended treatment effect brought about the observed improvement as suggested in the following study:

A controlled clinical trial of a new postoperative recovery program for posthysterectomy care was performed by randomizing 100 women postsurgery to a standard ward and 100 women to a special care ward equipped with experimental beds and postoperative exercise equipment and staffed by extra nurses. Women on the special care ward were discharged with an average length of stay of only 7 days compared to 12 days for women randomized to the regular ward. The results were statistically significant. The investigators concluded that the new postoperative recovery program resulted in a substantially reduced length of stay.

Before concluding that the experimental beds and postoperative exercise made the difference, do not forget that extra nurses were also required. The investigator's interest in early discharge and the availability of the extra nurses may have been the cause of the early discharge rather than the beds and exercise. In an unblinded study such as this one, it is possible that the effect of observation itself helped to bring about the observed effect. Although even a well-performed controlled clinical trial may not definitively establish that the treatment caused the improvement, for practical purposes controlled clinical trials satisfy the definition of *efficacy*.

Extrapolation

Patients included in most randomized controlled clinical trials are chosen because they are the type of patients most likely to respond to the treatment. In addition, considerations of geography, investigator convenience, and patient compliance are usually of paramount importance in selection of a particular group of patients for an investigation. Pregnant patients, the elderly, the very young, and those with mild disease are usually not included in controlled clinical trials unless the therapy is specially designed for their use. In addition to these selection factors that are under the control of the investigator, other factors may lead to entry of a unique type of patient group into controlled clinical trials. Every medical center population has its own referral patterns, location, and socioeconomic patterns. A patient population referred to the Mayo Clinic may be quite different from one drawn to a local county hospital. Primary care health maintenance organization (HMO) out-patients may be very different from the hospital subspecialty clinic out-patients. These characteristics, which may be beyond the investigator's control, may still affect the types of patients included in a way that may affect the results of the study.

The fact that the group of patients included in controlled clinical trials is different from a group of patients whom clinicians might treat with the new therapy often creates difficulty in extrapolating the conclusions to patients seen in clinical practice. This does not invalidate the result of a controlled clinical trial; however, it does mean the clinician must use care and judgment when adopting the results to clinical practice.

Thus despite the power and importance of controlled clinical trials, the process of extrapolation is still largely speculative. The use of convenient or chunk samples in controlled clinical trials makes it imperative that clinicians who wish to apply the study results examine the nature of the study institutions and the study patients. Clinicians should assess whether their own setting and patients are comparable to those in the study. If they are not comparable, the reader should ask whether the differences limit the ability to extrapolate from the study.

Patients and study centers involved in an investigation may be different from the usual clinical setting in many ways. For instance,

1. Patients in an investigation are likely to be carefully followed up and very compliant. Compliance and close follow-up may be critical to the success of the therapy.

2. Those in the study may have worse prognoses than the usual patients seen in clinical practice. For this reason the side effects of the therapy may be worth the risk in the study patients, but the same may not be true for patients seen in another clinical setting.

3. The study centers may have special skills, equipment, or experience that maximize the success of the new therapy. This may not be true when the therapy is used by those without experience with those techniques.

Despite a clear demonstration of a successful therapy using a controlled clinical trial, clinicians must be careful to take into account these types of differences in extrapolating to patients seen in their own clinical practices. Controlled clinical trials are capable of assessing the efficacy or benefit of treatment performed on a carefully selected group of patients treated under the ideal conditions of an experimental study. They must be used carefully when trying to assess the effectiveness of treatment as employed in usual clinical care. Thus well-motivated and conscientious physicians providing usual care with usual facilities probably will not be able to match the results obtained in controlled clinical trials.

Controlled clinical trials, at their best, are capable only of assessing the benefit or treatment under current conditions. Not infrequently, however, the introduction of a new treatment can itself alter current conditions and produce secondary or dynamic effects. Clinical trials have a limited ability to assess the secondary effects of treatment. This is especially true for those effects that are more likely to occur when the therapy is widely applied in clinical practice. Imagine the following study:

A new drug called "Herp-Ex" was shown to have efficacy in a controlled clinical trial. It was shown to reduce the frequency of attacks when used in patients with severe recurrent herpes genitalis. It did not, however, cure the infection. The investigators were very impressed with the results of the study and advocated its use for all individuals with herpes genitalis.

If Herp-Ex is approved for clinical use, several effects may occur that may not have been expected on the basis of a controlled clinical trial. First the drug would most likely be widely used extending its use beyond the indications in the original trial. Those with mild attacks or those presenting with first episodes would most likely also receive the therapy. The efficacy shown for recurrent severe attacks of herpes genitalis may not translate into effectiveness for uses that extend beyond the original indications. Second, the widespread use of Herp-Ex may result in strains of herpes that are resistant to the drug. Thus long-term efficacy may not match the short-term results. Finally, the widespread use of Herp-Ex and short-term success may reduce the sexual precaution taken by those with recurrent herpes genitalis. Thus over time the number of cases of herpes genitalis may actually increase despite or because of the short-term efficacy of Herp-Ex.

Controlled clinical trials are our fundamental tools for assessing the efficacy of therapy. When carefully used, they serve as a basis for extrapolations about the effectiveness of therapy in clinical practice. Controlled clinical trials, however, are not specifically designed to assess the safety of therapy. Prior to using a treatment as part of a controlled clinical trial, animal studies and limited human research are performed to help rule out frequent or severe effects of the treatment.

Rare and long-term effects, however, are not well assessed either before or during a controlled clinical trial.

Safety of therapy is more difficult to assess than efficacy. This is especially true for rare but serious side effects. The heart of the problem stems from the large number of individuals who need to receive the treatment before one is likely to observe rare but serious side effects.

The number of exposures required to ensure a 95% probability of observing at least one episode of a rare side effect is summarized in the *Rule of Three*. According to the Rule of Three, to have a 95% chance of observing at least one case of penicillin anaphylaxis, which occurs about 1 time per 10,000, one needs to treat 30,000 individuals. If one wishes to be 95% certain to observe at least one case of aplastic anemia from chloramphenicol, which occurs about 1 time per 50,000 uses, one would need to treat 150,000 patients with chloramphenicol. In general terms, the Rule of Three states that in order to be 95% sure one will observe at least one case of a rare side effect, one needs to treat approximately three times the number of individuals in the denominator.*

These numbers demonstrate that controlled clinical trials cannot be expected to detect many rare but important side effects. To deal with this dilemma, we often rely on animal testing. High doses of the drug are usually administered to a variety of animal species on the assumption that toxic, teratogenic, and carcinogenic effects of the drug will be observed in at least one of the animal species tested. This approach has been helpful but has not entirely solved the problem.

Long-term consequences of widely applied preventive treatments may be even more difficult to detect. Diethylstilbestrol (DES) was used for many years to prevent spontaneous abortions. It took decades before investigators noted greatly increased incidence of vaginal carcinoma among teen-aged girls whose mothers had taken DES.

It is only in clinical practice that a great number of patients are likely to receive the therapy. Therefore, in clinical practice we are likely to observe these rare but serious side effects. Alert clinicians and clinical investigators have been the mainstay of our current "post marketing surveillance." We currently have no organized systematic approach for detecting rare but serious side effects once a drug is released for clinical use. The FDA must rely on the reports received from practicing physicians. Thus clinicians need to be careful to remember that FDA approval should not be equated with complete safety or even with clearly defined and well-understood risks.

---

* These numbers assume there is no spontaneous or background incidence of these side effects. If these diseases occur from other causes, the numbers needed are even greater.

Controlled clinical trials are central to our current system for evaluating the efficacy of drugs and procedures. They represent a major advance. However, as clinicians reading the medical literature, we must understand their strengths and limitations. We must be prepared to draw our own conclusions about the application of the results to our own patients in our own settings. We must also recognize that controlled clinical trials can provide only limited data on safety and effectiveness of the therapy being investigated.

CHAPTER 12

Flaw-Catching Exercises: Controlled Clinical Trials

The following exercises are designed to test your skills in applying the principles of controlled clinical trials. Read each flaw-catching exercise, then write a critique pointing out the types of errors that occur in each component of the uniform framework.

BLOOD SAFE—A NEW TREATMENT TO PREVENT AIDS: EXERCISE NO. 1

An investigator believed he discovered an improved method for protecting the blood supply from the danger of spreading acquired immunodeficiency syndrome (AIDS) by killing the virus in the transfused cells. His method required treating all transfusion recipients with a new drug called "Blood Safe." At the time of his discovery, the rate of transmission of AIDS via blood transfusions was 1 per 100,000 transfusions.

Having gained approval to study this drug in humans, the investigator set out to design a controlled clinical trial for the initial use of the drug. He designed a study in which a random sample of all blood transfusion recipients in a major metropolitan area were asked whether they wished to receive the drug within 2 weeks after their blood transfusion.

The study enrolled 1,000 study group individuals who accepted the therapy. An additional 1,000 individuals who refused Blood Safe were used as the control group. Control group individuals had received an average of three blood transfusions compared to 1.5 for the average individual receiving Blood Safe. The investigators were able to obtain a follow-up human immunodeficiency virus (HIV) blood test on 60% of those receiving Blood Safe and 60% of those who refused approximately 1 month after their date of receiving a blood transfusion.

Those performing the follow-up blood testing were not aware of whether the patient received or did not receive Blood Safe. The investigator found that one patient in the study group converted to HIV antibody–positive within 1 month following treatment with Blood Safe. In the control group, two individuals converted.

The investigator did not find any evidence of side effects due to Blood Safe during the 1-month follow-up period. The investigator concluded that the study established that Blood Safe was effective and safe. He advised administration of Blood Safe to all blood transfusion recipients.

CRITIQUE: BLOOD SAFE—A NEW TREATMENT TO PREVENT AIDS

Study Design

The investigator intended to conduct a controlled clinical trial. Controlled clinical trials are best suited to assessing the efficacy of a therapy once a defined dose and method of administration have been developed during initial studies on humans. They are not well suited to the initial human investigations.

The risk of AIDS from blood transfusions at the time of the study was 1 per 100,000, a very low risk. Controlled clinical trials, which aim to reduce an already low risk, require a very great number of individuals. Many hundreds of thousands or even millions of individuals would be required to properly conduct a controlled clinical trial when the risk, without the treatment, is 1 per 100,000. A study of this size does not have adequate statistical power. In other words, this study would not be able to demonstrate statistical significance for this therapy, even if Blood Safe were capable of substantially reducing the incidence of AIDS due to blood transfusions, for instance from 1 per 100,000 to 1 per 1,000,000.

Assignment

The investigator identified a random sample of patients comparable to those who might receive an effective therapy. Random selection is not a requirement of controlled clinical trials, but it does make extrapolation to those in the sampled population who are not included in a controlled clinical trial more reliable.

The investigator did not randomize patients to the study group and the control group. The control group consisted of those who refused administration of Blood Safe. This is not an ideal control group, for those who refused to participate may be different from those who agreed to participate in a number of ways related to the potential for acquiring HIV infection. Randomization as opposed to random selection is considered a critical characteristic of a controlled clinical trial. Therefore, this study is not truly a controlled clinical trial.

Assessment

Those who assessed the outcome of this study were not aware of whether the patient had received Blood Safe. This blind and objective assessment helps prevent bias in the assessment process. The lack of blinding in the assignment process, however, means that patients were aware of whether they received Blood Safe. This may have had an effect on the outcome of the study if, for instance, those who received Blood Safe believed they were protected from acquiring AIDS.

The investigators assessed HIV antibody status 1 month after the patients received a transfusion. This is too early to adequately assess whether an individual actually will convert to an HIV antibody–positive status.

The great number of study and control patients who were lost to follow-up is an important assessment problem despite the fact that the percentages lost were equal in both groups. When the number of adverse outcomes is low, those lost to follow-up become especially important. Individuals lost to follow-up may disproportionately experience side effects or develop symptoms despite therapy.

Analysis

The investigator did not report statistical significance testing or confidence limits. If he had, he would not have been able to demonstrate statistical significance. This is not surprising since a single additional case of HIV infection would have made the outcome in the study group and control group equal.

The confidence interval in this study would be very wide, indicating that the results of this study are compatible with no difference or even a difference in the opposite direction.

The greater number of blood transfusions among those who refused Blood Safe may be a confounding variable that should be taken into account through an adjustment as part of the analysis. The number of blood transfusions is a confounding variable since the number of transfusions is different in the two groups and the number of transfusions is related to the risk of developing HIV infections secondary to blood transfusions.

Interpretation

The previous study design, assignment, assessment, and analysis problems mean that the study must be interpreted with great care.

The result of statistical significance testing and confidence intervals would imply that this difference in HIV infections between the study and control groups could be due to chance.

The risk of developing an HIV infection from blood transfusion in the absence of administration of Blood Safe is so small that other means of acquiring the AIDS infection may be much more likely. Therefore, any difference between a study group and a control group cannot automatically be attributable to Blood Safe. The difference in HIV infections may be due to differences between the study and control groups in other risk factors for AIDS. No data are presented that deal with these factors, which may be far more important risk factors than blood transfusions.

Extrapolation

Even if Blood Safe were shown to have efficacy in the prevention of transfusion-associated HIV infections, one could not draw conclusions about the effectiveness or safety from this study.

Controlled clinical trials can draw conclusions about the efficacy of therapy under the ideal conditions of an investigation. Effectiveness implies that the therapy has benefit under the usual conditions of clinical practice.

Using Blood Safe in clinical practice would imply administering Blood Safe to very great numbers of individuals. Thus rare but serious side effects are of importance. Despite the absence of side effects among those who received Blood Safe, rare but serious side effects may still occur. The Rule of Three states that if a serious side effect occurs once per 1,000 uses, then 3,000 individuals must be observed to be 95% sure of observing at least one case of the side effect.

In extrapolating from controlled clinical trials to use of a therapy in clinical practice, one must at a minimum consider the following:

1. Whether the study establishes the efficacy of therapy under ideal conditions
2. If individuals in the study are similar to those who will receive therapy
3. If known safety hazards or the possibility of rare but serious side effects not observed in controlled clinical trials outweigh the potential benefits

At times it may also be important to consider the cost of the treatment as compared to other options.

EXERCISE NO. 2: INFLUENZA VACCINE

A new vaccination for influenza was being tested in a randomized clinical trial. Participants were chosen for the study group by randomly selecting 1,000 families from a list of families who volunteered for the trial. In the 1,000 families, all 4,000 family members were given the vaccination. As a control group, the investigators randomly selected individuals from the telephone directory and offered them placebo vaccinations until 4,000 had accepted. In comparing the study and control groups, investigators found that the study group had an average age of 22 years versus an average age of 35 years for the control group. The study group was twice as likely to own a thermometer as the control group, but otherwise they were quite similar when compared on a long list of variables.

During the influenza season the following winter, each individual was instructed to see a study physician for any fever that occurred so that the possibility of influenza could be clinically evaluated. Study group subjects were assigned to one clinic and control group subjects to another. In their follow-up evaluation, the investigators gained the cooperation of 95% of the study group and 70% of the control group. The investigators found that the control group had 200 cases of influenza per 1,000 persons vaccinated and followed up versus 4 cases per 1,000 persons not vaccinated. They concluded that the new treatment cut the risk of influenza to 2% of its previous rate. The investigators recommended applications of the new treatment to the general population in order to eliminate 98% of the deaths due to influenza from this particular strain of virus.

CRITIQUE: EXERCISE NO 2

Study Design

The investigators failed to define what particular study sample they were using to try out the new therapy. It is not clear whether they were trying it out on families or individuals, on one age group or all age groups, on volunteers or the general population.

Assignment

In randomized clinical trials, investigators randomize and ideally blindly assign volunteers to either a control group or a study group. In this instance, all the volunteers were placed in the study group and given the experimental treatment. A separate sample was then developed to produce the control group. Therefore randomization and blind assignment were not performed.

Giving all members of a family the new vaccine produces the possibility that a partially successful treatment will appear almost fully effective. If the risk to a particular family member is reduced, the risk of exposure to influenza for the other family members will be greatly reduced since family exposure is an important source of transmission. Thus two factors favor the vaccinations: reduced exposure and increased immunity.

The investigators used a different population for selecting the new control group. By selecting names from the telephone book, the investigators limited their control sample to individuals listed in the telephone directory. This method did not result in a control group comparable to those receiving the treatment, particularly where children were concerned. Children are likely to be heavily represented in a population of families but not in the telephone directory.

Even if a random sample of a population is performed, a possibility exists that the study and control groups will not have an equal distribution of attributes potentially related to susceptibility to influenza. The age differences between the study and control groups (which might be expected from the method of assignment) need to be taken into account. The difference in frequency of thermometer ownership, even if it occurred by chance, is an important difference since it could affect the recognition of fever. An increased recognition of fever is likely to result in an increased diagnosis of influenza. Remember that random selection of subjects for a randomized clinical trial is a desirable but not a usual feature. Randomization, however, is essential since it is the hallmark of a randomized clinical trial.

Assessment

The method the investigators chose for assessment of influenza is not likely to be valid. Influenza is difficult to diagnose specifically, and no standard criteria are presented in the study for its diagnosis, such as culturing the virus. In addition, volunteers are likely to have a different threshold of illness before seeking medical care than nonvolunteers; this factor coupled with the decreased thermometer ownership by control group subjects could have influenced the number of diagnoses of influenza that were made. The fact that study and control group subjects were followed at different clinics suggests that blinding was not present. This may have affected the frequency of diagnosis of influenza.

Finally, unless follow-up is complete, the possibility exists that those lost to follow-up actually had either a better or a worse outcome than those who can be traced. A large proportion of the control group in the study was lost to follow-up, which may have affected the validity of assessment of outcome. In general, the assessment of outcome in this study was not valid.

Analysis

Since the study and control groups differed in their age distribution, and age is a frequent factor influencing susceptibility, it is important to adjust the data for the effects of age. This could be accomplished by comparing the influenza attack rate of individuals of the same age to see if the differences between vaccinated and unvaccinated individuals remained the same. In addition no statistical significance test was applied to see whether the differences found were likely if no true differences exist in the larger populations.

Interpretation And Extrapolation

The failure of this study to meet minimum standards for assignment, assessment, and analysis means that the study must be interpreted with great care. Many explanations other than a causal relationship can explain the reduced number of diagnoses of influenza in the study group.

Extrapolation to other populations requires convincing proof of a relationship among those in the study. Proof of a causal relationship was lacking in this study. Even if a relationship was established, one cannot extrapolate from influenza attack rates to death rates. The study, however, was not concerned with death rates and provided no evidence that the death rates were different in the two populations.

Despite the fact that the investigation had a great number of study design problems and the investigators extrapolated far beyond their data, it is important to note the magnitude of the effect that the study group had. A 98% reduction in the number of cases of influenza represents a very large effect. This finding needs to be examined closely despite the poor design of the investigation. It is often difficult but important to separate the quality of the therapy from the quality of the investigation.

PART 2

Testing a Test

CHAPTER 13

Introduction to Testing a Test

Medical diagnosis may be regarded as an attempt to make adequate decisions using inadequate information. Thus the uncertainty that is inherent in medical diagnosis stems from the need to make diagnoses based on uncertain data. The diagnostic tools used in medicine have been regarded traditionally as means of reducing the uncertainty in diagnosis. However, to successfully use diagnostic tests, one must appreciate not only how tests reduce uncertainty but also how they describe and quantitate the uncertainty that remains.

Historically, the diagnostic tools available were largely limited to a medical history and physical examination. These are still powerful diagnostic tools. Today however, in addition to conventional methods, a massive array of ancillary technology, properly and selectively employed, can provide the thoughtful clinician with precise diagnoses. Learning if and when we should apply each element of the history, physical examination, and ancillary technology constitutes the essence of the practice of diagnostic medicine.

Today's emphasis on cost-conscious quality requires that physicians understand the fundamental principles of diagnostic tests: which questions they answer and which they do not, which tests increase the diagnostic precision and which merely increase the cost.

To paraphrase Will Rogers, physicians traditionally have believed that nothing is certain except biopsy and autopsy. However, even these gold standards for diagnosis may miss the mark or be performed too late to help. A knowledge of the principles of diagnostic tests helps to define the extent of diagnostic uncertainty as well as to increase certainty. Knowing how to live with uncertainty is a central feature

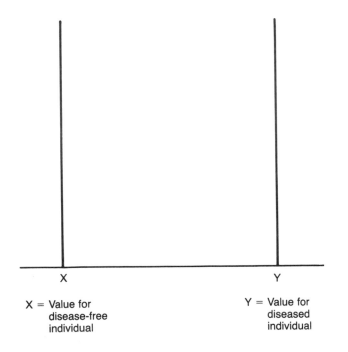

X = Value for
    disease-free
    individual

Y = Value for
    diseased
    individual

FIGURE 13-1   *Conditions required for a perfect diagnostic test.*

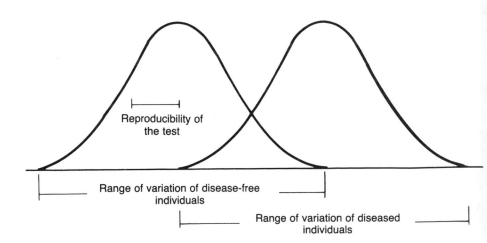

FIGURE 13-2   *The three types of variations that affect diagnostic testing.*

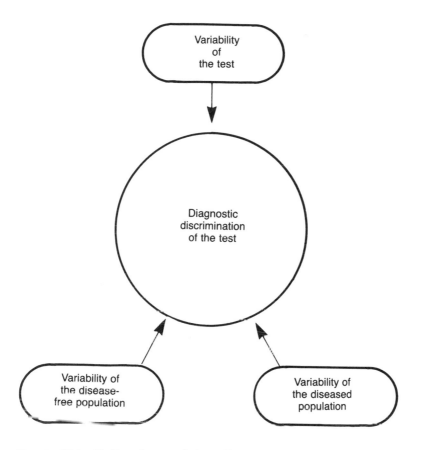

FIGURE 13-3   *Uniform framework for testing a test.*

of clinical judgment: The skilled physician has learned when to take risks to increase certainty and when to simply tolerate uncertainty.

The fundamental principle of diagnostic testing rests on the belief that individuals with disease are different from individuals without disease and that diagnostic tests can distinguish between these two groups. Diagnostic testing, to be perfect, would require that (1) all individuals without the disease under study have one uniform value on the test, (2) all individuals with the disease under study have a different but uniform value for the test, and thus (3) all test results are consistent with the results of the diseased or those of the disease-free group (Fig. 13-1).

If this were the situation in the real world, then one perfect test could distinguish disease from health, and the physician's work would be merely to order the "right" test. The real world, for better or worse, is not so simple. None of these three conditions is usually present. Variations exist within each of the three basic factors: the tests, the group with disease, and the disease-free group (Fig. 13-2).

The assessment of diagnostic tests is largely concerned with describing the variability of these three factors and thereby quantitating the conclusions that can be reached despite or because of this variability.

The variability, reproducibility, and accuracy of the test itself are discussed in Chapter 14. In Chapter 15 the variability of the disease-free population is reviewed and assessed using the concept of a range of normal. In Chapters 16 and 17 the variability of the diseased population and its relationship to the disease-free population are quantitated using the concepts of sensitivity, specificity, and predictive value. These concepts are outlined, and the errors in their implementation are illustrated. Flaw-catching exercises then provide an opportunity to apply these principles to the evaluation of diagnostic tests.

As with analyzing a study, it is helpful to have an overview, a generalized framework for evaluating a test. This framework is depicted in Figure 13-3, which illustrates the variability that exists in tests, in the disease-free population, and in the diseased population. It also emphasizes that these variations must be studied and incorporated into any assessment of the diagnostic utility of a test.

CHAPTER 14

Variability of the Test

A perfect test would produce the same results every time it was conducted under the same conditions. In addition, its measurement would reflect exactly the phenomenon that the test intended to measure. In other words, a perfect test would be completely reproducible and completely accurate. Let us first define these terms and see how they are used.

Reproducibility is the ability of a test to produce consistent results when repeated under the same conditions and interpreted without knowing the first test's results. Several factors, however, may affect the reproducibility of a test:

1. The patient and laboratory conditions under which the test is repeated may not be the same.
2. The test may be affected by variations in interpretation from person to person. This effect is known as *interobserver variability*.
3. The test may be affected by variations in interpretation by the same person at different times. This effect is known as *intraobserver variability*.

In assessing the method for performance of the test, researchers must be sure that the technical and biologic conditions for performance are identical when the test is repeated. Failure to follow this precaution results in the error illustrated in the following example:

The reproducibility of a test for serum cortisol levels was evaluated by drawing two samples from the same individuals. The first sample was drawn at 8 A.M. and the second at noon. Methods for performance were identical, and interpretation was performed without knowledge of the results of the first test. This method was applied to 100 randomly selected individuals. The authors found that, on the average, the second test results were twice the level found in the same individual's first test. They concluded that the large variation indicated that the test was not reproducible.

Remember that reproducibility is the ability of the test to produce nearly the same results when conducted under the same conditions. In this example, the investigators did not repeat the test under identical conditions. A natural cycle occurs in the individual's cortisol level throughout the day. By drawing blood at 8 A.M. and again at noon, the investigators were sampling at two different times in the cycle. Even if this test were completely reproducible when performed under identical laboratory conditions, the different conditions of the patients under which it was administered would produce quite different results.

Failure to perform a repeat test without knowledge of the first test's result may allow the second reading to be influenced by the first reading as illustrated in the following example:

An investigator, studying the reproducibility of a urinalysis, asked an experienced laboratory technician to read a urinalysis sediment, to leave the slide in place, and then to repeat the reading in 5 minutes. The investigator found that the reading, performed under the same conditions, produced perfectly reproducible results.

In this example, the technician knew the results of the first test and was likely to have been influenced by the first reading when rereading the urine sample 5 minutes later. A measure of reproducibility requires that the second measurement be performed without knowing the results of the first measurement. Thus, the technician should not have known the results of the previous reading.

Even if interpreters are unaware of their own or other previous readings of the test, the possibility of individual variation exists, which can introduce error when comparing test results. Whenever judgment is involved in the interpretation of a test, there is room for inter- and intraobserver variations. Two radiologists frequently interpret the same x rays differently; this is known as interobserver variation. An intern may interpret an electrocardiogram differently in the morning from his or her middle-of-the-night reading of the same test. This is known as intraobserver variation. These variations do not in themselves destroy the usefulness of a test. They do require that the physician be alert to the constant probability of variation in interpretation. Inconsistencies of technique or interpretation contribute to some extent to the variability in most tests. It is necessary therefore to have criteria to judge how much variability can be tolerated.

In general, it is important that the variability of the test be much smaller than the range of variability due to biological factors. Thus the extent of variation in the test should be small compared to the range of normal for the test (see Chap. 15).

It is important to distinguish reproducibility from accuracy. The *accuracy* of a test is its ability to produce results that are close to the true measure of the anatomical, physiological, or biochemical phenomenon. Accuracy of a test requires that a test be reproducible but it also requires that the result is free of a systematic tendency to differ from the true numerical value in one particular direction. When shooting at a target, the bull's-eye may be missed because of scattering of the bullets on all sides of the bull's-eye. There also may be a tendency to place all bullets slightly to one side. To be perfectly accurate and hit the bull's eye every time, there must be reproducibility, thus eliminating the scatter. There must also be lack of bias or a tendency to shoot to one side. Therefore, an accurate test is free of random or chance, as well as systematic errors or biases. A test may be very reproducible yet quite inaccurate, reproducing results that are far from the true value. The following example illustrates a test of good reproducibility but poor accuracy, exemplifying the difference between reproducibility and accuracy:

A study was conducted on 100 patients undergoing surgery for navicular fractures. Each of the study patients had two independently interpreted x rays. Both x rays were negative for navicular fracture within the week after their initial injury. The authors concluded that the radiologists had been negligent in missing these fractures.

Navicular fractures frequently are not diagnosed correctly or at all by x ray at the time of injury. Anatomically the fracture is there, but the x ray is not usually capable of detecting its presence until evidence of healing appears. Therefore, it may not be the negligence of the radiologists so much as the inaccuracy of the test that was used. Repeating the x-ray tests confirmed the reproducibility of the negative results obtained by the radiologists: It is not possible to recognize early navicular fractures by x ray. *Accuracy* means that the test will produce a result that is close to the true anatomic, physiologic, or biochemical value. Since x rays are not always an accurate reflection of the anatomy, the test was at fault, not the eye of the radiologists.

A test may be quite accurate when employed in a scientific study, but it may lose its accuracy when applied in the clinical setting. It is helpful to think of two types of accuracy: (1) experimental accuracy—the accuracy of the test when applied under careful study conditions, and (2) clinical accuracy—the accuracy of the test when applied under real clinical conditions. The difference between the two concepts is illustrated in the following example:

In a university hospital, a study was conducted of 500 patients on a 3-day, low-fat diet. It showed that the fat content in stools collected for 72 hours after the diet successfully separated those patients with malabsorption from those without it. An identical study protocol administered to 500 out-patients failed to identify successfully the presence of malabsorption. The authors of the out-patient study concluded that the in-patient results were incorrect.

The performance of a test is usually assessed under ideal experimental conditions. The field condition under which it is employed often may be less than ideal. A 72-hour stool collection after 3 days on a low-fat diet may be very difficult to collect on an out-patient basis. The fact that the out-patient data do not agree with the in-patient data may merely reflect the realities of the field conditions. Accuracy is a required property of a good test. Accuracy alone, however, does not ensure that the test will be valid or useful for diagnosis. *Valid* implies that the test is an appropriate measurement for the question being addressed. A very reproducible and accurate measure of lung size may provide little information that is valid or useful for diagnosis. To establish the diagnostic utility of a test, we need to assess how well the test separates those who are free of the disease from those with the disease.

Before we attempt to determine how well a test separates those with disease from those without disease, let us first turn our attention to how we measure those without disease using the concept of the range of normal.

CHAPTER 15

The Range of Normal

Disease-free human populations are subject to inherent biological variations. One need only to walk down the street to appreciate the differences among people. Individual height, weight, and color cover a span that reflects the wide, but not unlimited, variations that can occur among healthy individuals.

In a world with complete information, we would know what an individual's measurement on a particular test should be. This would enable us to compare the results of a test to the individual's expected level. In reality we rarely know what an individual's level should be, so we are forced to compare one individual's level with those of other individuals who are believed to be free of disease. To perform this comparison, we use a *range of normal*. The range of normal is thus a necessary evil built on the assumption that a particular individual should be similar to other individuals.

The concept of a range of normal is an effort to measure and quantify the range of values that exist among individuals believed to be disease-free. A range of normal can be derived for any measurement in which multiple possible numerical values exist for disease-free individuals. These include measurements of physical examination characteristics such as blood pressure, liver size, and heart rate, or laboratory values such as hematocrit, sedimentation rate, or creatinine. Although the range of normal measurements are often wide, the concept does not include all those who are free of disease. It intentionally leaves out 5% of the individuals who are believed to be disease-free in order to create a range of normal that is wide enough to describe most disease-free measurements but not so wide as to include all possible numerical values. If the range of normal included the measurements on all individuals without disease, it would be extremely wide, so wide in fact that it would not generally be useful for separating those with disease from those who are disease-free. The range of normal is descriptive not diagnostic. It describes disease-free individuals; it does not diagnose disease. Values outside the range of normal may be the result of chance variation, physiologic changes unassociated with disease, or pathologic changes secondary to disease.

DEVELOPING THE NORMAL RANGE

The range of normal values might be developed as follows:

1. The investigator locates a particular group of individuals who are believed to be disease-free. This group is known as the *reference group*. These individuals are frequently medical students, hospital employees, or other easily accessible volunteers. They are usually merely assumed to be disease-free though in some circumstances they may have undergone extensive testing and follow-up to ensure that they are disease-free.

2. The investigator then performs the test of interest on all the individuals in the reference group.

3. The investigator next plots the distribution of test measurements among this disease-free reference group.

4. The investigator then calculates a range of normal that includes the central 95% of the reference population. Strictly speaking, the range of normal includes the mean or average measurement plus or minus the measurements within two standard deviations from the mean. Unless there is a reason to do otherwise, the investigator generally chooses the central part of the range so that 2.5% of disease-free individuals have measurements above and 2.5% of disease-free individuals have measurements below the range of normal.

To illustrate the method for developing the range of normal, imagine that investigators have measured the heights of 100 male students in a medical school and found numerical values that looked like those in Figure 15-1. The investigators would then choose a range of normal that includes 95 of the 100 medical students. Unless they had a reason to do otherwise, they would use the middle part of the range so that the range of normal for this reference group would be from 60 to

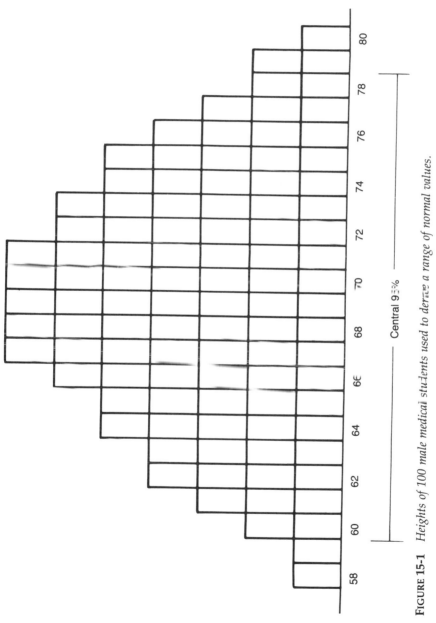

Central 95%

FIGURE 15-1 Heights of 100 male medical students used to derive a range of normal values.

78 in. Individuals outside this range may not have any disease; they may simply be healthy individuals who are outside the range of normal.

BASIC PRINCIPLES

Let us look first at the implications of those principles of the range of normal and then illustrate the errors that can result from failure to understand these implications.

1. By definition, 5% of a group will have a measurement on a particular test that lies outside the range of normal. Thus "abnormal" and "diseased" are by no means synonymous. The more tests that are performed, the more individuals there will be who are outside the range of normal on at least one test. Taking this proposition to its extreme, one might conclude that a "normal" person is anyone who has not been investigated sufficiently. Despite the absurdity of this proposition, it emphasizes the importance of understanding that the definition of the range of normal intentionally places 5% of disease-free individuals outside the range of normal. Thus the term *outside normal limits* must not be equated with disease.

2. Values that lie within the range of normal do not ensure that the individual is disease-free. The ability of the range of normal on a test to discriminate disease from disease-free individuals varies from test to test. Unless the test is perfect in ruling out disease—and few tests are—some individuals with the disease will have measurements of the test that lie within normal limits.

3. Changes within normal limits may be pathologic. Since the range of normal includes a wide range of numerical values, an individual's measurement may change considerably and still be within normal limits. For instance, the range of normal for the liver enzyme AST is 8 to 20 U/L, the range of normal serum potassium may vary from 3.5 to 5.4 mEq per L, and the range of normal uric acid may range from 2.5 to 8.0 mg per 100 ml. It is important not only to consider whether an individual's measurement lies within normal limits but also to consider whether the individual's test result has changed over time. The concept of a range of normal is most useful when no historical data are available for a comparison of individual patients. When previous results are available, however, they should be taken into account.

4. The range of normal is calculated using a particular group of patients or reference population who are believed to be disease-free.

Therefore, when applying a particular range of normal to an individual, one must ascertain whether this individual has a reason to be different from the reference population used to calculate the range of normal. For instance, if men are used to obtain a range of normal hematocrit, this range of normal cannot necessarily be applied to women, who generally have lower hematocrits.

5. The range of normal must not be confused with the desirable range. The range of normal is an empirical measurement of the way things are among a group of individuals currently believed to be disease-free. It is possible that large segments of the community possess test results that are higher than ideal and may be predisposed to develop a disease in the future.

6. The upper and lower limits of the range of normal can be altered for diagnostic purposes. The range of normal includes 95% of those who do not have a particular condition or disease. It does not require, however, that the same number of disease-free individuals will have test results below the range of normal as have test results above the range of normal. There is some room for scientific judgment to determine where the upper and lower margins of the range of normal should be set. Where to set the limits depends on what a researcher or clinician desires to accomplish by using the test.* For instance, suppose that most of the individuals with a disease are found to have measurements nearer the upper limits of the range of normal for the test. If the investigator is willing to lower the upper limits of the range of normal, a larger proportion of those with the disease can be expected to have test results above the range of normal. Then, however, the investigator pays the penalty (or makes the trade-off) of labeling a larger proportion of the disease-free population as outside the range of normal. At times it may be worth paying this penalty, especially when it is important to detect as many individuals as possible with the disease or when the follow-up testing to clarify the situation is cheap and convenient. This trade-off is illustrated in Figure 15-2.

By shifting the range of normal to the left as in the range of normal No. 2, note that area B becomes smaller than in the range of normal No. 1, and that area A becomes larger. In other words, a decrease in the number of false-negatives leads to an increase in the number of false-positives, and vice versa. More persons with the disease are now identified as outside normal limits by the test. At the same time, more

---

* The level set for the range of normal defines the specificity of the test. This level may subsequently be adjusted to increase (or decrease) the specificity. Thus in actual use the range of normal has been adjusted whenever the specificity is not 95%.

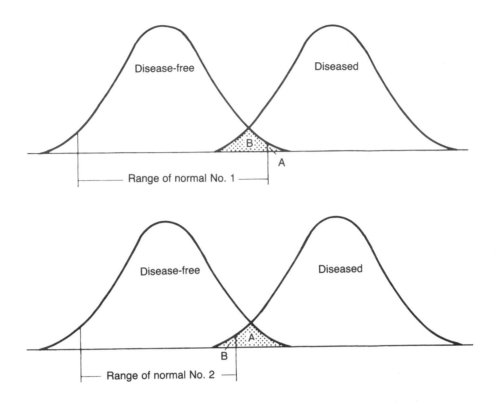

FIGURE 15-2   *Shifting the range of normal. False-positive, A: Individuals who are disease-free and who have values higher than the range of normal. False-negative, B: Individuals who have disease and who have values within the range of normal.*

individuals who are disease-free are classified as outside normal limits, therefore in range of normal No. 2 we are trading off more false-positive readings for less false-negative ones. How many false-positives and how many false-negatives the physician or medical system is willing to tolerate depends on ethical, economic, and political considerations as well as medical knowledge.

The following examples demonstrate errors that result from failure to apply each of these principles:

1. In a series of 1,000 consecutive health maintenance examinations, a series of 12 laboratory tests (SMA-12) was done on each patient even though no abnormalities were found on a medical history or physical examination. Five percent of the SMA-12s were outside the range of normal, a total of 600 "abnormal" tests. The authors concluded that these test results fully justified doing SMA-12s on all health maintenance examinations.

Let us look at the meaning of these tests results. A range of normal values, by definition, includes only 95% of those who are believed to be free of the condition. If a test is applied to 1,000 individuals who are free of a condition, 5% or 50 individuals will have test results outside the range of normal. If 12 tests are applied to 1,000 individuals without evidence of pathology, then on average 5% of 12,000 tests performed will be outside the range of normal. Five percent of 12,000 equals 600 tests. Thus, even if these 1,000 individuals were completely free of disease, one could expect 600 test results that are outside the range of normal. Those merely reflect the method of determining the range of normal. Test results outside the range of normal do not necessarily indicate pathology and do not by themselves justify doing multiple laboratory tests on all health maintenance examinations.

In considering the implications of test results, it is important to realize that all levels outside the range of normal do not carry the same meaning. Numerical values well beyond the limit of the range of normal may be much more likely to be caused by disease than numerical values that are near the borderlines of the range of normal. Test results nearer the limits of the range of normal are more likely to be due to variation of the test or to normal biologic variation. For instance, if the upper limits of male hematocrit are 52, then a value of 60 is more likely to be associated with disease than a value of 53.

2. One hundred chronic alcoholics underwent AST determinations to assess liver function. The majority were found to have AST results within the range of normal. The authors concluded that these alcoholics had well-functioning livers.

This example illustrates the difference between range of normal laboratory tests and the disease-free state. The fact that these individuals had laboratory tests within normal limits did not in and of itself establish that their livers were functioning properly since, on any one test, some diseased individuals will be within the range of normal. The poorer the capacity of the test to diagnose disease, the more individuals there will be with a disease who will have test results within the normal limits of the test. On certain tests individuals with a disease may not be distinguishable from disease-free individuals. Both groups may have test results mostly within the range of normal. This appears to have occurred for the AST results. The failure of the test to separate diseased from disease-free individuals indicates that the test had poor diagnostic discrimination, and it is not useful for diagnosis. This emphasizes the distinction between within the range of normal and disease-free.

Figures 15-3 to 15-5 illustrate three possible relationships between the disease-free and the diseased population. Figure 15-3 illustrates a

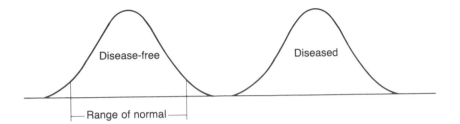

FIGURE 15-3   *A test with complete separation of populations results in perfect diagnostic discrimination.*

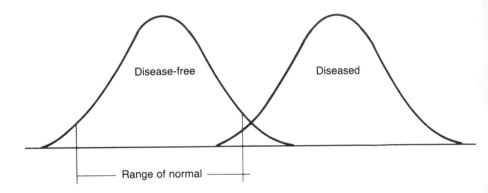

FIGURE 15-4   *A test with partial separation of the populations results in partial diagnostic discrimination.*

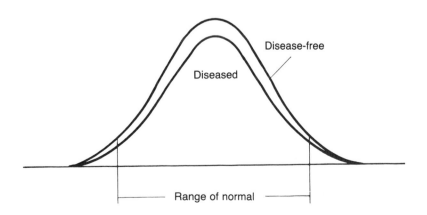

FIGURE 15-5   *A test with no separation of the populations results in no diagnostic discrimination.*

test that completely separates those with disease from those who are disease-free. The diagnostic discrimination of this test is perfect. Figure 15-4 illustrates the usual situation in which a test partially separates those with disease from those without disease. Figure 15-5 illustrates the situation in which a test has no diagnostic discrimination: Individuals with disease have the same test results as individuals without disease. In the AST example, the situation closely resembles Figure 15-5. Despite its utility in diagnosing many liver diseases, AST determination does not appear useful for diagnosing the chronic effects of alcohol on the liver. Thus despite the ability to calculate a range of normal for any test, the range of normal alone will not indicate whether the test will be useful in diagnosis. Measurements for individuals with a particular disease may be identical to those of the disease-free group or vice versa, indicating that the test is of no utility for diagnosing a particular disease.

3. Among 1,000 asymptomatic Americans with no known renal disease and with no abnormalities showing on urinalysis, the range of normal for serum creatinine were found to be 0.7 to 1.4 mg/dl. A 70-year-old woman was admitted to the hospital with a serum creatinine of 0.8 mg/dl and was treated with gentamicin. On discharge, she was found to have a creatinine value of 1.3 mg/dl. Her physician concluded that since her creatinine was within normal limits on admission as well as on discharge, she could not have had renal damage secondary to gentamicin.

The presence of a result within the normal range does not ensure the absence of pathology. Each individual has a disease-free measurement that may be higher or lower than the average measurement for individuals without disease. In this example, the patient increased her serum creatinine over 60% but still fell within the range of normal. The change in the creatinine measurement suggests a new pathologic process was occurring. It is likely that the gentamicin produced renal damage. When historical information is available, it is important to include it in evaluating a test result. Changes within the range of normal *may* be a sign of disease.

4. A group of 100 medical students was used to establish the range of normal values for granulocyte counts. The range of normal was chosen so that 95 of the 100 granulocyte counts were included in the range of normal. The range of normal granulocyte was determined to be 2,000 to 5,000. When asked about an elderly black male with a granulocyte count of 1,900, the authors concluded that this patient was clearly outside the range of normal and needed to be further evaluated to identify the cause of the low granulocyte count.

The range of normal is dependent on the disease-free reference population chosen; it is usually defined as the range around an average value, which includes 95% of the individuals in a particular reference population. However, the disease-free reference population used for determining a range of normal measurement may have different measurements from the group of individuals for whom one wants to use the test.

It is unlikely that there are many elderly black males among the group of medical students used to establish the range of normal. In fact, black males have a different range of normal granulocyte count from white males. Thus, the range of normal established for the medical students may not have reflected the range of normal applicable to this elderly black male. This man was probably well within the range of normal for an individual of his age, race, and sex. Since elderly black males are known to have their own range of normal, this must be taken into account when interpreting the test results.

5. The range of normal of serum cholesterol, as determined among 100 white American males aged 30 to 60 years, was found to be 200 to 300 mg/dl. A 45-year-old white American male was determined to have a serum cholesterol of 280 mg/dl. His doctor informed him that since his cholesterol was within normal limits, he did not have to worry about the consequences of high cholesterol.

A range of normal is calculated using data collected from a reference population currently believed to be disease-free. It is possible that the group used consists of many individuals whose results on the test are higher (or lower) than desirable. A result within the range of normal does not ensure that an individual will remain disease-free. It may be that American males as a group have higher-than-desirable cholesterol levels. If this is true, the patient with a cholesterol of 280 mg/dl may well suffer the consequences of high cholesterol. When research data are available strongly suggesting a range of desirable numerical values for a test, it is permissible to substitute the desirable range for the usual range of normal. Increasingly this is being done for serum cholesterol.

6. A study found that 90% of those with intraocular pressure greater than 25 mm Hg will develop visual defects secondary to glaucoma within the next 10 years. Twenty percent of those with pressures of 20 mm Hg will develop similar changes, and one percent of individuals with pressures of 15 mm Hg will develop defects. The authors concluded that performance on the test could be improved by setting the upper limits of normal at 15 mm Hg instead of 25 mm Hg since the test then could identify nearly everyone with the risk of developing visual defects (Fig. 15-6).

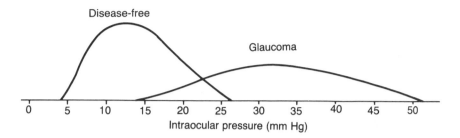

FIGURE 15-6   *Possible distribution of intraocular pressure for those with glaucoma and those who are disease-free.*

If 25 mm Hg is the upper limit of normal, then nearly everyone who will not develop glaucoma will be inside the range of normal, but a great number of individuals who will develop glaucoma will be included also within the normal range. On the other hand, if one sets the upper limits of normal at 15 mm Hg, very few individuals with glaucoma will be within the normal range, and a great number of individuals who will never develop glaucoma are outside the normal range.

The ability of a test to detect disease can be increased by altering the limits for the range of normal. If the limits are extended far enough, the test will include nearly everyone with the condition. Unfortunately, this attractive solution also labels an increased number of individuals as outside the range of normal who do not have and will not have a pathologic condition. By increasing the upper limits of normal, the investigators increased the ability to detect future disease but only by paying the price of following up on a greater number of individuals who are destined to remain disease-free. In determining where to set the upper limits, the following factors might be considered:

1. Vision loss from glaucoma is largely irreversible and may develop before it is apparent to the patient.
2. Treatment is generally safe but only partially effective in preventing progressive visual loss.
3. Follow-up is safe and involves little risk, but follow-up of a great number of individuals is time-consuming and costly, requiring multiple repeated examinations extending over long periods of time. Follow-up produces anxiety among those for whom it is required.

The trade-offs then are not simply medical. Additional social, psychologic, economic, and political considerations can all be incorporated into the decision of where to set the cut-off line. There may well be no correct answer. The only way out of this no-win situation may be to come up with a better test, one that has less overlap between those who will develop disease and those who will not.

The concept of a range of normal is an attempt to deal with the variability that exists among humans. An understanding of the utility and limitations of this concept is central to an understanding of diagnostic tests. The range of normal defines the numerical values found for 95% of a particular reference group who are believed to be disease-free individuals. The range of normal may not reflect the desirable level, and it does not take into account changes from previous test results.

The range of normal per se tells us nothing about the diagnostic utility of a test. Every test has a range of normal that may or may not help in distinguishing individuals with disease from those without disease. To determine the utility of a test in diagnosing disease, it is necessary to look at the test results for a group of individuals with a particular disease and to compare those values with the normal range of a disease-free group, as we do in Chapter 17. Before we can do this, however, we need to take a look at how we define those with disease.

CHAPTER 16

Defining Disease: The Gold Standard

Individuals with disease as well as disease-free individuals show a range of measurement on any test. The variability of individuals with disease may result from different severities of the disease or from differences in the individual's response to the disease. Despite this variability, it is essential to define a group of patients who definitely have the disease.

THE GOLD STANDARD

The test or criterion used to unequivocally define the disease is known as a *gold standard*. The gold standard may be a biopsy, an angiogram, a subsequent autopsy, or any other established test. The use of a gold standard to definitively identify those with the disease is a necessary prerequisite to examining the diagnostic utility of any new or unevaluated test. In other words, the usefulness of the new test rests on its comparison to the gold standard. Thus a new test is compared to an older and better established test (or tests) to determine if the new test can do as well as the previous gold standard. Notice it is assumed that, using the best of the older, established tests, it is possible to be 100% correct in making a diagnosis—the assumption being that it is impossible to invent a better mouse trap since you cannot do better than 100%. There might be a cheaper or more convenient mouse trap but, by definition, not one that catches more mice.

It may sound like a "catch-22" to claim that the only way to evaluate a new test's diagnostic ability is to assume that it is already possible to make perfect diagnoses. Unfortunately, this is the position we are in when evaluating a new test. We can ask only whether the test measures up to the best of the old tests, that is, the gold standard.

Despite the inherent limitation of our ability to initially evaluate a new test, time and repeated applications are on the side of the better mouse trap. Once applied in clinical practice, it may become evident that the new test actually predicts a subsequent clinical course better than the gold standard. It is even possible that eventually the new test will be accepted as the gold standard. Often, however, the problem is that definitive diagnosis is possible but is too dangerous or too late to be of maximum clinical benefit. In such instances, an adequate gold standard exists but not a clinically practical test. Under these circumstances, it is beneficial to determine that a new test measures up to the gold standard. Once again one must understand that the goal of assessing a test is limited to comparing it to the best available test. Thus one must be sure that the best available gold standard is being used. Let us see what can happen when the gold standard is less than ideal in the following example:

One hundred individuals, admitted to a hospital with "diagnostic Q waves" on their electrocardiograms (ECGs) and dying within 1 hour of admission, were autopsied for evidence of myocardial infarction (MI). The autopsy was used as the gold standard for MI. Autopsy revealed evidence of MI in only 10. The authors concluded that the ECG was not a useful method of making the diagnosis of an MI. They insisted on the gold standard of pathological diagnosis.

The utility of all diagnostic tests is determined by comparison to a gold standard test that has previously been shown by experience to diagnostically measure the characteristic under study. Autopsy diagnoses are frequently used as a gold standard against which all other tests are judged. At times, even an autopsy is a less-than-perfect measure of disease as illustrated in this example since the pathologic criteria for MI may take considerable time to develop. It is possible that the diagnostic Q waves on an ECG are a better reflection of an MI than pathological changes at autopsy. The investigator should be sure that the gold standard being used has in fact been shown to be the best available standard before using it as a basis for comparison.

Unfortunately, even the best available gold standards often do not unequivocally differentiate all those with the disease from those without it. Individuals with early or mild disease may not fulfill the gold standard criteria. Investigators are often tempted to include only those individuals who have clear-cut evidence of disease as measured by the gold standard. Despite the seemingly intellectual certainty that this provides, this may result only in a investigation of those with severe or far advanced disease. This danger is illustrated in the next example:

An investigator studied the ability of urine cytology to diagnose bladder cancer as compared with unequivocal biopsy-diagnosed cases of invasive bladder cancer that fulfilled the gold standard diagnosis. The cytological examination detected 95% of those with bladder cancer. However, when applied in clinical practice, urine cytology only detected 10% of those with bladder cancer.

By using cases of advanced invasive bladder cancer, the investigators have eliminated those with early or equivocal disease. Thus we should not be surprised to find that the test fails to perform as well in clinical practice as it performed when compared to a clear-cut gold standard test.

As tempting as it is to study only individuals with clear-cut disease, it is deceptive to draw conclusions about the utility of a test when using only individuals with severe or far advanced disease. When assessing the diagnostic discrimination of a test, it is important to ask whether the best available gold standard was used to define those with disease. However, it is also important to ask whether those with the disease spanned the entire spectrum of individuals who have the disease. We must recognize that at times it is impossible to satisfy both of these goals simultaneously.

Even if these conditions are fulfilled, one must appreciate that the goal of testing a test is limited to determining whether the test being studied is as good as the established gold standard. The methods used do not address the possibility that the new test might be better than the gold standard.

CHAPTER 17

Diagnostic Discrimination of Tests

It is now possible to derive measurements of the ability of a test to discriminate between those with disease and those who are disease-free. In doing so, it is important to remember the following three prerequisites for such an assessment:

1. Variability of the test: A measurement of the reproducibility of the test finding. The range of variability should be relatively small in comparison to the range of normal
2. Variability of the disease-free population: A determination of the range of normal values for the test
3. Definition of the gold standard: Identification of groups of individuals who definitely have and those who do not have the disease as defined by the gold standard

SENSITIVITY AND SPECIFICITY

The traditional measures of the diagnostic value of a test are its *sensitivity* and *specificity*. They measure a test's diagnostic discrimination compared to that of the gold standard, which by definition has a sensitivity of 100% and a specificity of 100%. Sensitivity and specificity have been chosen as measures because they are inherent characteristics of a test that should be the same when the test is applied to a group of patients in whom the disease is rare or to a group of patients in whom the disease is frequent.* Thus they provide measurements

---

* This may not be strictly true if the proportion of early disease changes along with the frequency of disease. A test may have different sensitivity and specificity for early versus more advanced disease.

of the diagnostic discrimination of a test that should be the same regardless of the probability of disease before performing the test. The stability of the sensitivity and specificity allows researchers in Los Angeles, Paris, or Tokyo to apply the same diagnostic test and expect similar results despite their very different populations. Sensitivity and specificity also allow researchers and clinicians to directly compare the performance of one test to another.

Sensitivity measures the proportion of those with the disease who are correctly identified by the test. In other words, it measures how sensitive the test is in detecting the disease. It may be helpful to remember sensitivity as *positive in disease* (PID). Specificity measures the proportion of those without the disease who are correctly called disease-free by the test. Specificity can be thought of as a *negative in health* (NIH).

Notice that sensitivity and specificity tell us only the proportion or percentage of those with or without a disease who are correctly categorized. These measures do not predict the actual number of individuals who will be correctly categorized. The actual number of individuals will depend on the frequency of the disease in the group being tested.

Sensitivity and specificity are useful measures because they allow readers and researchers to obtain the same results when assessing a test on groups of patients with different frequencies of the disease. Sensitivity and specificity, however, may have different numerical values when they are obtained using a group of patients with early stages of a disease compared to the sensitivity and specificity obtained in a group of patients with more advanced disease.

Let us first outline the mechanism for calculating sensitivity and specificity and then outline the implications and limitations. In calculating the sensitivity and specificity of a test in comparison to the gold standard, researchers proceed in the following manner:

1. The investigators choose the gold standard to be used in defining diseased individuals.

2. The investigators next choose one group of patients that the gold standard indicates has the disease and another group that the gold standard indicates does not have the disease. In implementing this criterion, it is important to know whether investigators included a representative group of individuals with and without the disease. In other words, do the individuals chosen represent a full spectrum of individuals who have the disease and who are disease-free, or do they represent only the two ends of the spectrum? In choosing these individuals, it has become common practice to select as many diseased individuals as disease-free individuals defined by the gold standard. This 50-50 split, however, is not necessary.*

3. Researchers must now use the test being investigated to categorize all study individuals as positive or negative. To do this for tests whose results are presented as numerical values, they must use the range of normal. For instance, if most individuals with the disease have values above the range of normal, then investigators use the upper end of the range of normal as the cut-off point. Investigators test all individuals with the new test and classify them positive or negative.

4. The investigators have now classified each patient as diseased or disease-free according to the gold standard and positive or negative by the test. They then can calculate the number of individuals for whom the test and the gold standard agree and the number of individuals for whom they disagree and display their results as follows:

TEST	GOLD STANDARD DISEASED	GOLD STANDARD DISEASE-FREE
Positive	a = Number of individuals diseased and positive	b = Number of individuals disease-free and positive
Negative	c = Number of individuals diseased and negative	d = Number of individuals disease-free and negative
	a + c = Total number of diseased individuals	b + d = Total number of disease-free individuals

5. Finally, investigators apply the definitions of sensitivity and specificity and calculate their values directly.

---

* The 50-50 split provides the greatest statistical power for a given sample size. However, we rarely see statistical significance tests applied to assessments of diagnostic tests since the sample size is usually small and thus the statistical power is usually low.

$$\text{Sensitivity} = \frac{a}{a + c} = \begin{array}{l}\text{The proportion of those with disease}\\\text{according to the gold standard who are}\\\text{labeled positive by the test}\end{array}$$

$$\text{Specificity} = \frac{d}{b + d} = \begin{array}{l}\text{The proportion of those who are}\\\text{disease-free according to the gold standard}\\\text{who are labeled negative by the test}\end{array}$$

To illustrate this procedure using numbers, let us imagine that a new test is performed on 500 individuals who have the disease according to the gold standard and 500 individuals who are disease-free by the gold standard. We can now set up the 2 × 2 table as follows:

TEST	GOLD STANDARD DISEASED	GOLD STANDARD DISEASE-FREE
Positive	a	b
Negative	c	d
	500	500

Now suppose that 400 of the 500 individuals with the disease are labeled positive by the test and that 450 of the 500 disease-free individuals are labeled negative by the test. One can now fill in the 2 × 2 table.

TEST	GOLD STANDARD DISEASED	GOLD STANDARD DISEASE-FREE
Positive	400	50
Negative	100	450
	500	500

Sensitivity and specificity can now be calculated.

$$\text{Sensitivity} = \frac{a}{a + c} = \frac{400}{500} = 0.80 = 80\%$$

$$\text{Specificity} = \frac{d}{b + d} = \frac{450}{500} = 0.90 = 90\%$$

A sensitivity of 80% and a specificity of 90% symbolize a diagnostic test, although not ideal, is in the range of many tests we use in clinical medicine to diagnose disease.

Notice that the test has been applied to a group of patients in which 500 have the disease and 500 are disease-free individuals as defined by the gold standard. This division of 50% with the disease and 50% disease-free is the usual division chosen for study. The sensitivity and specificity would have been the same regardless of the number of diseased and disease-free patients chosen. One way to convince yourself of the truth of this important principle is to look at how the sensitivity and specificity are calculated, that is,

$$\text{Sensitivity} = \frac{a}{a + c} \text{ and specificity} = \frac{d}{b + d}$$

Notice that a and c, which are necessary to calculate sensitivity, are both contained in the left-hand column of the chart. Similarly b and d, which are necessary to calculate specificity, are both contained in the right-hand column of the chart. Thus the total number of individuals in each column does not really matter since sensitivity and specificity each relate only to the division of patients who are within a single column.

Once the sensitivity and specificity have been calculated, it is possible to work backward and fill in the table when different numbers of diseased and disease-free patients, as defined by the gold standard, are used. This time let us assume that there are 900 disease-free individuals and 100 individuals with disease. In other words, this is the situation in which 10% of the individuals being tested have the disease. Thus the average individual has a 10% probability of having the disease even before the test is performed.

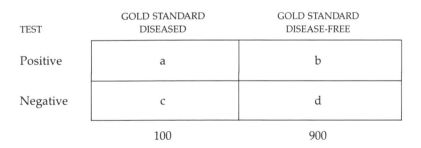

TEST	GOLD STANDARD DISEASED	GOLD STANDARD DISEASE-FREE
Positive	a	b
Negative	c	d
	100	900

Now let us apply the sensitivity and specificity measures as previously determined.

Sensitivity equals 80%; therefore, 80% of those with the disease will be correctly labeled as positive (80% of 100 = 80). And 20% of those with the disease will be incorrectly labeled as negative (20% of 100 = 20).

Specificity equals 90%; therefore, 90% of those who are disease-free will be correctly labeled as negative (90% of 900 = 810. And 10% of those who are disease-free will be incorrectly labeled as positive (10% of 900 = 90).

The following 2 × 2 table can now be constructed.

	10% PREVALENCE	
TEST	GOLD STANDARD DISEASED	GOLD STANDARD DISEASE-FREE
Positive	80	90 False positives
Negative	20 False negatives	810
	100	900

This is a situation in which 10% of the patients under study have the disease as defined by the gold standard; therefore, we can say that in this group of patients, the true probability of having the disease is 10%.

Let us now compare this table to the one developed when sensitivity and specificity were first calculated. Since we used 500 diseased and 500 disease-free individuals, we were actually using a group of patients with a 50% probability of having the condition.

	50% PREVALENCE	
TEST	GOLD STANDARD DISEASED	GOLD STANDARD DISEASE-FREE
Positive	400	50 False positives
Negative	100 False negatives	450
	500	500

Notice that with our original 50-50 division (i.e., 50% prevalence,) 100 individuals were falsely labeled negative, and 50 were falsely labeled positive. In the group of patients with 10% prevalence, however, 20 individuals were falsely labeled negative, and 90 individuals were falsely labeled positive. The change in numbers is solely the result of the difference in relative frequency of disease or prevalence in the two groups of patients studied (50% versus 10%). Notice that in the 10% prevalence example there are actually more positives who are disease-free (90) than positives who have the disease (80).

This may be surprising in light of the relatively high sensitivity and specificity. However, it illustrates a principle that must be recognized in applying the concepts of sensitivity and specificity. Thus, despite the fact that sensitivity and specificity are not directly influenced by the relative frequency or prevalence of the disease, the actual number of individuals who are falsely labeled positive and falsely labeled negative is dependent on the relative frequency of the disease.

Now let us look at an even more extreme situation, the case where only 1% of the group being tested has the disease. This is typical of the situation when we are screening a group of individuals who have risk factors for a common disease but no clinical evidence of disease. This situation may be charted as below:

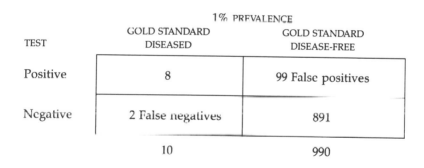

	1% PREVALENCE	
TEST	GOLD STANDARD DISEASED	GOLD STANDARD DISEASE-FREE
Positive	8	99 False positives
Negative	2 False negatives	891
	10	990

In this screening situation we have again used the same test with 80% sensitivity and 90% specificity. This time, however, there are 8 true-positives and 99 false-positives or over 12 false-positives for every true-positive. Thus sensitivity and specificity alone do not provide a complete indication of how useful a result will be in diagnosing a disease for a particular individual. As clinicians and users of diagnostic tests, we need to know more than a test's sensitivity and specificity. We need to be able to address the clinical questions: What is the probability of disease if the test is positive? What is the probability of no disease if the test is negative? Before we can answer these questions we must ask what is the probability of disease before the patient receives the test. This *pretest probability* along with the test's sensitivity and specificity allows one to calculate measures known as the *predictive value of the test*.

PREDICTIVE VALUE OF POSITIVE AND NEGATIVE TESTS

As previously discussed, the major advantage of sensitivity and specificity as measures of a test is that they are not directly dependent on
the prevalence or pretest probability of the disease. This advantage is
particularly useful for articles in the medical literature. Sensitivity and
specificity, however, have shortcomings in answering two clinically
important questions: If the test is positive, how likely is it that the
individual has the disease? If the test is negative, how likely is it that
the individual does not have the disease? These questions are of
practical concern to clinicians.

The measures that answer these queries are known as the *predictive
value.*

> Predictive value of a positive test = The proportion of those
> with a positive test who
> have the disease

> Predictive value of a negative test = The proportion of those
> with a negative test who
> do not have the disease

The terms *prevalence* and *predictive value* are used in research articles
dealing with groups of individuals. Fortunately, counterpart terms
are used in clinical practice where the clinician deals with one individual at a time. Clinically the *prevalence* of the condition means the same
as the best estimate of the probability of disease before performing the
test. In clinical terms, prevalence is known as *pretest* probability. *Predictive value* means the same as the probability of the disease being
present (or absent) after obtaining the results of the test. Thus predictive values can be thought of clinically as *posttest probability.* If the
terms *prevalence* and *predictive value* are confusing to you, substitute
the concept of *probability of the disease* before and after the test.

As a rough guide to interpreting the numbers, it may be helpful to
use the following approximate pretest probabilities:

> 1% = Pretest probability of those with risk factors for a common
> disease but without any symptoms
> 10% = The pretest probability when a disease is unlikely but possible
> clinically and the clinician wishes to rule it out
> 50% = The pretest probability when there is considerable uncertainty but
> the clinical presentation is compatible with the disease
> 90% = The pretest probability when the disease is very likely clinically
> but the clinician wishes to rule it in using a diagnostic test

Using 2×2 tables, let us illustrate how to calculate the predictive
value. When calculating predictive value, remember we do so for one
particular prevalence or pretest probability of the disease.

TEST	GOLD STANDARD DISEASED	GOLD STANDARD DISEASE-FREE
Positive	a = Number of individuals diseased and positive	b = Number of individuals disease-free and positive
Negative	c = Number of individuals diseased and negative	d = Number of individuals disease-free and negative

a + b = Total number of positives   c + d = Total number of negatives

The following formulae are used for calculating the predictive value of a positive test and the predictive value of a negative test.

Predictive value of a positive test $= \dfrac{a}{a+b}$ Proportion of those with a positive test who actually have the disease (as measured by the gold standard)

Predictive value of a negative test $= \dfrac{d}{c+d}$ Proportion of those with a negative test who actually do not have the disease (as measured by the gold standard)

Let us now calculate these values starting with pretest probabilities of 90%, 50%, 10%, and 1%. Remember that the number of positives and negatives will be different for each prevalence of the disease.

90% PRETEST PROBABILITY

TEST	GOLD STANDARD POSITIVE	GOLD STANDARD NEGATIVE
Positive	720	10
Negative	180	90

900   100

90% Pretest Probability

Predictive value of a positive test $= \dfrac{a}{a+b} = \dfrac{720}{730} = 98.6\%$

Predictive value of a negative test $= \dfrac{d}{c+d} = \dfrac{90}{270} = 33.3\%$

Using the same procedure the remaining predictive values are:

50% Pretest Probability

$$\text{Predictive value of a positive test} = \frac{a}{a + b} = \frac{400}{450} = 88.9\%$$

$$\text{Predictive value of a negative test} = \frac{d}{c + d} = \frac{450}{550} = 81.8\%$$

10% Pretest Probability

$$\text{Predictive value of a positive test} = \frac{a}{a + b} = \frac{80}{170} = 47.1\%$$

$$\text{Predictive value of a negative test} = \frac{d}{c + d} = \frac{810}{830} = 97.6\%$$

1% Pretest Probability

$$\text{Predictive value of a positive test} = \frac{a}{a + b} = \frac{8}{107} = 7.5\%$$

$$\text{Predictive value of a negative test} = \frac{d}{c + d} = \frac{2}{891} = 99.8\%$$

For a test with a sensitivity of 80% and a specificity of 90%, these data can be summarized as follows:

Pretest probability	1%	10%	50%	90%
Predictive value of a positive test	7.5%	47.1%	88.9%	98.6%
Predictive value of a negative test	99.8%	97.6%	81.8%	33.3%

Thus these calculations of predictive values have important clinical implications. They indicate that the probability of a disease being present or absent after obtaining the results of a test is dependent on the best possible estimate of the probability of disease made before performance of the test. When the probability of disease is moderately high before performance of the test, for example 50%, even a negative test like the one used in our example leaves an 18.2% (100–81.8%) probability that the disease is present. When the probability of disease is relatively low before performance of the test, for instance 10%, even a positive test leaves a 52.9% (100%–47.1%) probability that the disease is absent.

The situation is even worse when the same test is used as a screening test. For instance we might be testing a group of individuals who have a risk factor for the disease but only a 1% probability of having active disease. As we can learn from our example with a 1% prevalence or pretest probability of disease, when we apply our test with 80% sensitivity and 90% specificity to this group of individuals, those with a positive test will still have only a 7.5% probability of having the disease. That is what a predictive value of a positive test of 7.5% means. Failure to understand the effect of pretest probability on predictive value can lead to the following error:

A new, inexpensive test for lung cancer was evaluated by applying it to a group of 100 individuals with lung cancer and 100 individuals with no evidence of cancer. A positive test was shown to have a predictive value of 85%, that is, 85% of those with a positive test have lung cancer. The authors concluded that this test was well suited for screening the general population, since 85% of those with a positive test will have lung cancer.

The predictive value of a positive test is the percentage of those with a positive test who have the disease. The predictive value depends on the prevalence of the disease in the group of individuals tested. In evaluating a test, it is often applied to individuals, half of whom are known to have the disease. In this example, the test was applied to a group in which 50% of the individuals had the disease (100 with lung cancer, 100 without lung cancer). Thus, the prevalence or pretest probability of the disease in the test group was 50%. The lower the pretest probability of the disease, the lower the predictive value of a positive test will be.

In the community, even among those who smoke cigarettes, the prevalence of lung cancer will be much lower than 50%; therefore, the predictive value of a positive test when applied to an average individual from the community, even one with risk factors for lung cancer, will be far below 85%. The ability of a positive test to predict disease changes dramatically when the test is used on groups of individuals with different probabilities of having the disease. A positive test may have a high predictive value in one group of patients; however, in another group of patients with a different prevalence or prior probability of disease, the same positive test may have a much lower predictive value. Such a test may be useful for diagnosis in a group of patients with a high suspicion of disease, but it will be useless for screening a general community with low suspicion of disease.

COMBINING TESTS

In clinical practice and in the increasingly frequently published research literature of decision analysis, researchers look at the effects of combining tests. Two tests can be combined in two basic ways: in series or in parallel.

The use of two tests in series may lead to a diagnosis using the following testing strategy:*

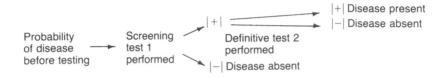

Using two tests in series, test No. 2 is performed only on those individuals who are positive on test No. 1. The probability of disease after the results of both tests are positive is calculated by regarding the predictive value of a positive test after test No. 1 as same as the probability of disease before performing test No. 2. Serial tests allow physicians to rule out disease using fewer tests although serial testing often takes more time.† If both tests are performed on everyone either test may come first.** However, if only positives receive further testing, using the test with highest sensitivity first assures maximum disease detection.

The strategy of using tests in parallel requires that both tests be performed, and the probability of disease is considered after performance of both tests as depicted in the following chart.‡

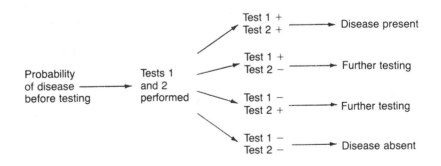

---

*   Figure from R. K. Riegelman, and G. J. Povar (eds.), *Putting Prevention into Practice.* Boston: Little, Brown, 1988.
†   Testing in series can also be helpful if both tests have a low specificity.
** This assumes that the tests are independent of each other. In other words, it assumes that the second test will have the same sensitivity and specificity regardless of the results of the first test.
‡   Figure from R. K. Riegelman, and G. J. Povar (eds.), *Putting Prevention into Practice.* Boston: Little, Brown, 1988.

This parallel strategy works well when neither test has a particularly high sensitivity but each picks up a different type of disease. One test might detect early disease, whereas the other might detect more established disease. Alternatively one test may detect rapidly developing or aggressive disease, whereas the second test may detect more indolent or slowly progressive disease.

Both serial and parallel strategies assume that the second test provides additional information above and beyond that provided by the first test. When this is not the case, both strategies perform less well than expected. For instance, imagine the following use of a parallel strategy:

Breast examination and thermography were studied as parallel tests for detecting breast cancer. It was found that breast examination had a sensitivity of 40% and thermography had a sensitivity of 50%. Using the two together, the study found that only 50% of the breast cancer was detected by one or the other tests. The investigators where surprised since they had expected to be able to detect most of the breast cancer cases.

Combining the use of breast examination with thermography adds little to the use of either test alone since neither test detects early disease. The results of the tests may give us the same basic information, and thus knowing the results of one test is all we need. Tests of this type work poorly together whether used in parallel or in series.

Thus when designing a diagnostic strategy for testing, we need to learn more than sensitivity and specificity: We need to know whether the tests measure different or independent phenomena. We also need to learn what type of disease the tests miss. Do they fail to detect early disease or slowly progressive disease?

CHAPTER 18

Summary: Testing a Test

Our framework for testing a test requires us to evaluate the test itself using the concept of reproducibility and accuracy, the variation of those without disease using the concept of the range of normal, and those with disease as measured by the gold standard. This information is then combined to give an assessment of the diagnostic discrimination of the test as measured by sensitivity, specificity, and predictive values.

The variability of a test is measured by its reproducibility, that is, the test is repeated under the same conditions. Repetitions of the test are then interpreted without knowledge of the first test results. Reproducibility does not in itself ensure the accuracy of a test. A reproducible test can reproduce inaccurate results if a bias occurs in one direction. Some variation is expected, but it should be much smaller than the biological variation as measured by the range of normal.

Variability among individuals without the disease is measured by the range of normal. The range of normal often includes only 95% of those who are believed to be disease-free. The range of normal is dependent on the reference group chosen. Remember that the range of normal is merely descriptive of the way things are among supposedly disease-free individuals. It is not diagnostic: Outside normal limits does not equal diseased; within normal limits does not equal disease-free; change within the range of normal may be pathologic; and within normal limits is not necessarily the same as desirable. The borderline for the range of normal may be adjusted, thereby altering the specificity, but the price paid in the number of false-positives and false-negatives must be taken into account. Finally, in using the concept of the range of normal to define a disease-free group of individuals, unequivocal limits must be set in order to determine which patients are positive and which patients are negative as measured by the test.

The group of patients with the disease is defined by the gold standard, which is the generally accepted best available method for diagnosing the disease. In defining those with the disease, it is desirable to include individuals with the same type of pathology as will be encountered in the clinical application of the test.

Having determined that a test is reproducible, having defined both a positive and a negative test using the range of normal and—using the gold standard—having identified a group of diseased and disease-free individuals, one is ready to assess the diagnostic discrimination of a test.

When the test under study is applied to individuals who are identified as being diseased or disease-free by the gold standard, the sensitivity and specificity of the test are calculated by comparing individuals' results on the test with their results according to the gold standard. Since the gold standard is assumed to have 100% or perfect diagnostic discrimination, the test under study will usually fall short of the gold standard; this is true even if the test is inherently better than the gold standard since any discrepancy will be decided in favor of the gold standard.

Sensitivity measures the proportion of those with the disease—as diagnosed by the gold standard—who are correctly identified as having the disease by the test under study. Specificity measures the proportion of those without the disease—measured by the gold standard—who are correctly identified by the test as being disease-free. Sensitivity and specificity are important since they are in theory independent of the prevalence or pretest probability of the disease in the group of individuals being studied. This allows comparison to test results obtained on different patient groups. Tests can be compared directly to one another using the measures of sensitivity and specificity. It is important to recognize, however, that sensitivity and specificity may be different in early stages of a disease compared with later stages.

Sensitivity and specificity do not answer this clinical question: What is the probability of the disease if the test is positive or if it is negative? The predictive value of a positive test tells us how well the test rules in disease in a particular clinical situation. The predictive value of a negative test tells us how well the test rules out the disease in a particular clinical situation. The predictive values, unlike sensitivity and specificity, are dependent on the prevalence or pretest probability of the disease.

Clinically, this means that the clinician should make the best possible estimate of the probability of disease before performing the test.

The predictive value then tells the clinician the probability of the disease being present after performance of the test. The clinician should be careful not to extrapolate the predictive value from one clinical setting to another. A test that is very useful for diagnosing the disease in the presence of symptoms may be nearly useless for screening asymptomatic individuals.

Tests may be combined in series or in parallel. When two tests are used in series, the second test is performed only if the first test is positive. Testing in series may enable a diagnosis to be made utilizing fewer tests. Tests may be used in parallel when neither test has an adequately high sensitivity. This testing strategy works well when the two tests detect different types of the disease such as early and late or aggressive and intolerant disease. In this situation use of tests in parallel helps ensure that a higher percentage of individuals with the disease will be detected. Obtaining maximum benefit from either of these strategies requires that the results of the two tests measure different phenomena or pick up disease at a different stage in its development.

QUESTIONS TO ASK IN TESTING A TEST

The following checklist of questions to ask should help to reinforce the principles involved in testing a test.

1. Inherent properties of a test
   a. Reproducibility. Do multiple repetitions of the test under the same conditions produce nearly identical results?
   b. Accuracy: Are the test results close to the true measure of the anatomic, physiologic, or biochemical phenomena?
   c. Clinical accuracy: Under conditions of actual clinical performance, has the test been shown to produce measurements that are close to the experimentally derived measurement?
2. Biologic variation: The concept of the range of normal and variability of disease-free individuals
   a. Has a range of normal been properly obtained to include a defined percentage often 95% of those believed to be free of disease?
   b. Has outside the range of normal been distinguished from diseased?
   c. Has inside the range of normal been distinguished from disease-free?
   d. Is the reference group used generally applicable or are there identifiable groups with different ranges of normal?

e. Have those who applied the test recognized that the range of normal is a description of a presumably disease-free group and that changes within the range of normal for any one individual may be pathologic?
f. Has the range of normal been distinguished from desirable?
g. Have the investigators justified moving the range to accomplish specific diagnostic goals?
3. Variability of the diseased individuals
   a. Have the investigators chosen the best available gold standard for defining which patients have the disease under study?
   b. Have the investigators included a broad enough cross-section of those with the disease to produce a realistic range of measurements for those with the disease?
4. Diagnostic discrimination: Distinguishing diseased from disease-free individuals
   a. How well does the test identify those with disease? How high is its sensitivity? How often is it positive in disease?
   b. How well does the test identify those without disease? How high is its specificity? How often is it negative in health?
   c. Has it been recognized that despite the fact that in theory sensitivity and specificity are not affected by the posttest probability of disease, they may be different for early versus more advanced disease?
   d. Have the sensitivity and specificity of the test been distinguished from the predictive value of a positive test and the predictive value of a negative test?

LABORATORY TESTS

Let us examine a few of the basic laboratory tests used in clinical medicine to assess their accuracy, reproducibility, range of normal, and diagnostic discrimination.

Hematocrit

Accuracy And Reproducibility

The hematocrit is a measurement of the percentage of the total blood composed of packed red blood cells. Routine hematocrits are measured by either the finger stick method of assessing capillary blood or the venipuncture method. Both methods can accurately measure the relative quantity of red cells to total blood, but reproducibility of the techniques requires attention to technical detail. Capillary blood can be expected to have a hematocrit about 1 to 3% lower than venous blood. Excessive squeezing of the finger tip can milk out extra plasma and falsely lower the hematocrit. When anemia is severe, the finger stick measurement is less accurate.

In assessing the accuracy with which the hematocrit assesses the physiological status, remember that relative and not absolute red cell mass is being tested. Misleading results are possible when dehydration or diuresis lowers the plasma volume. Individuals with reduced plasma volume may present with hematocrits above the range of normal. These are normal variants but may be confused with polycythemia (pathologically elevated hematocrit).

Range Of Normal

The range of normal levels of the hematocrit are different for men and women. This is generally recognized and reported by laboratories as separate ranges of normal for men and women. Less often recognized are different levels of normal for different stages of pregnancy, different ages, and persons living at different altitudes. The hematocrit usually falls during pregnancy beginning somewhere between the third to the fifth month. Between the fifth and eighth month, a reduction of 20% compared to previous levels is not unusual. The hematocrit generally rises slightly near term and should return to its previous level by 6-weeks postpartum.

Age has a pronounced effect on hematocrit, especially among children. The range of normal on the first day of life is 54 ± 10 (i.e., the range of normal is 44 to 64). By the fourteenth day, the range is 42 ± 7. By 6 months the normal range is 35.5 ± 5. The average hematocrit gradually increases through the teen-aged years, with the average reaching 39 between 11 and 15 years of age. Adult ranges of normal are, for men, 47 ± 5, and for women, 42 ± 5.

Low barometric pressure has a pronounced effect on the range of normal hematocrits. Native residents who live at high altitudes have generally higher hematocrits. The range of normal at about 4,000 ft, for instance, is 49.5 ± 4.5 for adult men and 44.5 ± 4.5 for adult women.

The range of values for normal hematocrits is quite wide. Thus if an individual begins near the upper end of the normal range, as much as one-fifth of the red cell volume may be lost before anemia can be demonstrated by a low hematocrit. Comparisons with previous hematocrits are important in assessing the development of anemia. For any one individual, the hematocrit is physiologically maintained within quite narrow limits. Thus changes in hematocrit are a better diagnostic measure than evaluation of a single observation.

Diagnostic Discrimination

When evaluating the hematocrit, one must be aware of the method by which the hematocrit responds to acute bleeding. During the acute bleed, whole blood is lost, and the remaining blood initially will approximate the original hematocrit. It may require 24 hours or more before compensation occurs through increase in the plasma volume. Only after compensation does the hematocrit fully reflect the extent of blood loss. Failure to recognize this phenomenon leads to false-negatives in recognizing acute bleeding.

The body is frequently able to compensate for slow blood loss or destruction. Therefore, despite an elevated reticulocyte count, patients with slow bleeding or hemolysis may not demonstrate anemia. If one expects to detect diseases predisposing to blood loss or destruction by ordering a hematocrit, then one will find a relatively great number of false-negatives. Conditions like B-thalassemia and glucose-6-phosphate dehydrogenase (G-6PD) deficiency often present as compensated anemia with a low-normal or normal hematocrit. False-positives may occur among those with expanded plasma volume as a normal variant. From another aspect, these individuals reflect the fact that for any range of normal, some individuals without disease will have values outside the normal range.

Blood Urea Nitrogen And Serum Creatinine

Accuracy And Reproducibility

The blood urea nitrogen (BUN) and serum creatinine are automated tests that are obtained quite reproducibly. BUN and serum creatinine reflect the serum accumulation of unexcreted urea nitrogen and creatinine, thus they reflect the inability of the kidney to excrete these substances. When used as measures of renal function, they attempt to assess the glomerular filtration rate. They most accurately reflect glomerular filtration rate in the presence of substantial renal impairment. The kidneys ordinarily have considerable reserve function, thus substantial loss of function, one kidney for instance, may occur without increased accumulation of BUN and creatinine. Only after a 50% or greater loss of total glomerular filtration do the BUN and serum creatinine begin to accurately reflect glomerular filtration rate.

As glomerular filtration rate decreases further, the BUN and creatinine start increasing at faster and faster rates. The percentage increase in BUN and creatinine rather than the numerical change more accurately reflects the percentage loss in glomerular filtration rate once BUN and serum creatinine are clearly elevated.

When the creatinine is within the normal limits and one needs a more accurate assessment of glomerular filtration rate, it is possible to get a 24-hour urine for creatinine plus a simultaneous serum creatinine, and to calculate the creatinine clearance. Although this test has its own problems with reproducibility and range of normal, it is capable of detecting much smaller changes in glomerular filtration rate when the serum creatinine is not elevated.

Range Of Normal

The standard laboratory range of normal for BUN is approximately 10 to 20 mg/dl, and it is 0.6 to 1.4 mg/dl for creatinine. Using these ranges of normal requires an understanding of the factors that affect these levels in the absence of disease. BUN is a reflection of the protein status and hydration of a patient. Thus a patient's BUN can change substantially without indicating specific disease. Creatinine is a product of muscle and, as such, varies widely among disease-free individuals according to their muscle mass. Women generally have lower creatinine levels than men, and the elderly as a group have lower muscle masses and comparably lower serum creatinines. Despite these substantial differences, laboratories generally report creatinine levels as a single range of normal.

Creatinine as opposed to BUN varies less from day to day and month to month in response to nonrenal factors. Comparisons of creatinine with previous levels can often provide important information about renal status. A serum creatinine level of 1.3 for an elderly woman may reflect considerable loss of glomerular filtration rate especially if it has increased compared to previous determinations. The same level for a muscular young man may be stable and will give no indication of diminished glomerular filtration rate.

Diagnostic Discrimination

False-negatives for renal disease using the BUN and creatinine are very common, since as previously discussed, BUN and creatinine do not begin to rise until substantial loss of glomerular filtration has occurred. In addition, false-positives occur with both BUN and creatinine. BUN levels may be low in diseases that lead to malnutrition. Alcoholics, for instance, frequently have low BUN levels. BUN also reflects blood breakdown that occurs during rapid loss of blood into the gastrointestinal tract. These elevations of BUN are not strictly false-positives since they indicate disease other than renal disease. They are false-positives, however, if one is trying to assess glomerular filtration. Falsely elevated creatinine can occur in the presence of muscle disease. Again, these are not really false-positives, but they suggest a disease other than renal disease.

It is possible to use BUN and creatinine testing in parallel to help understand and localize the abnormalities. Ordinarily the ratio of BUN to creatinine is about 15 : 1. Elevation of BUN out of proportion to creatinine is suggestive of pre- or postrenal disease rather than intrinsic kidney disease. Thus dehydration generally will give a prerenal pattern of BUN elevated out of proportion to creatinine. Occasionally, one will find a postrenal disease such as prostate obstruction that also results in a BUN elevated out of proportion to creatinine. Thus the simultaneous or parallel use of BUN and creatinine is an example of a situation where use of two tests will produce more diagnostic information than use of either test alone since these tests measure different phenomena.

Uric Acid

Accuracy And Reproducibility

Uric acid levels in the blood can be measured reproducibly using automated techniques. There are several different methods, each of which gives slightly different levels. It is important to compare levels obtained by the same method. Automated techniques generally give slightly higher levels. Levels of uric acid can vary over short periods of time. Dehydration, for instance, can rapidly and significantly increase uric acid.

Uric acid blood levels accurately measure the uric acid in the serum. They do not, however, accurately assess all the important physiological parameters of uric acid. They are not an accurate gauge of total body uric acid. Crystalized and deposited uric acid, for instance, is not included in the serum measurement. With respect to the development of gout, crystalized and deposited uric acid is often the governing consideration. In addition, uric acid serum levels are only one factor affecting the excretion of uric acid. Some individuals without a high level of serum uric acid may excrete large quantities of uric acid, predisposing them to uric acid stones.

Range Of Normal And Diagnostic Discrimination

The range of normal values for uric acid is quite wide, with the range of normal varying from about 2 to 8 mg/dl in most laboratories, with some variation depending on the method used. A great number of individuals are found with values slightly above this range of normal and very few are found with values below this range. Very few individuals with values only slightly above this range develop gout. This has caused many physicians to argue that slightly high levels of uric acid should not be treated. They are really arguing that the upper range of normal should be increased so that the serum level of uric acid can better discriminate those who are predisposed to gout from those who are not.

Even at high levels of uric acid, the diagnostic discrimination is not good. False-positives occur frequently. Individuals with renal failure often have very high serum uric acid but rarely develop gout. Obviously, other factors besides the serum uric acid level determine the development of gout. In predisposed individuals, gout has been shown to develop at times when the uric acid blood levels are changing rapidly. Reductions as well as increases can precipitate gout. Individuals with gout frequently have uric acid serum levels within the range of normal when they present with gout. These cases are documented by the gold standard test, demonstration of birefringent crystals in the joint fluid, rather than by their serum level of uric acids. Those suspected of gout, but with levels of uric acid within normal limits during their acute attack, should be rechecked at a later time. Their uric acid levels then will often be increased, demonstrating the existence of a false-negative at the time of onset of gout.

Because of the weak association between serum uric acid and urine excretion, serum uric acid can be said to have poor diagnostic discrimination for uric acid stones. The number of false-positives and false-negatives would be very large if one used serum levels as the exclusive diagnostic criterion. Actual demonstration of uric acid stones is the most definitive method of diagnosis. Elevated 24-hour urine excretion of uric acid has been shown to predispose to uric acid stones. The association here, however, is not one to one either, since many other factors affect stone formation. A low urine volume and a low urine PH, in particular, are important predisposing factors increasing the frequency of uric acid stones.

Uric acid demonstrates several important principles applicable to diagnostic tests:

1. Even in the presence of an accurate and reproducible test that reflects the metabolic abnormality linked to disease, there may be

a low degree of association between serum level and the existence of pathology.

2. Serum levels as measured for uric acid and many other tests may not be a good reflection of total body levels, in particular, levels at the site of the pathology.

3. Serum levels may be least dependable at the time when they are needed most, at the onset of symptoms.

C H A P T E R 19

Flaw-Catching Exercises: Testing a Test

The following exercises are designed to evaluate your ability to apply the various principles used in *Testing a Test*. The exercises include a variety of errors, which have been illustrated in the hypothetical examples. Read each exercise, then write a critique pointing out the types of errors committed by the investigators. Compare your critique to the sample critique provided.

EXERCISE NO. 1: VARIABILITY OF THE DISEASED AND THE DISEASE-FREE POPULATIONS

Two investigations were conducted to evaluate the diagnostic utility of a new test for breast cancer. The test had previously been shown to have test results that varied by less than 1% when repeated under the same conditions and read by the same interpreter.

In the first study, the investigators chose 100 women with metastatic breast cancer and 100 healthy women without any signs of breast disease. Results of the test for the healthy women were 30 to 100 mg/dl. Results for breast cancer patients ranged from 150 to 200 mg/dl. Since this test perfectly separated the two groups, the investigators concluded that it could be considered an ideal test for diagnosing breast cancer and should immediately be applied to screening all women.

In a second study using the same test, another investigator compared 100 newly diagnosed breast cancer patients with 100 patients with benign breast disease. The cancer patient's results ranged from 70 to 200 mg/dl, whereas the patients with benign breast disease ranged from 40 to 180 mg/dl. The authors of this study noted the tremendous overlap between the two groups and concluded that the test was worthless.

A reader of these studies could not understand how two respected investigators could produce such inconsistent results. He concluded that there must have been errors in reporting the test results.

CRITIQUE: EXERCISE NO. 1

To review these studies, it is helpful to organize the discussion by using the concepts of the variability of the test, the variability of the disease-free group, and the variability of those with the disease.

Variability Of The Test

Reproducibility is the measure of variability of the test. The study states that the test had previously been shown to have had only a 1% variation when conducted under the same conditions by the same interpreter. A measure of reproducibility requires repeat performance of the test to demonstrate that the second results are not influenced by the results of the first test. The same interpreter performed the repetition of the test results, thus it is possible that he or she was influenced by the initial results. If this were true, then the reproducibility might be poorer than was previously reported. In the rest of this discussion, however, let us assume that the authors are correct in believing that the test is reproducible.

Variability Of The Disease-Free Group

The first study used healthy patients and found a range of numerical values from 30 to 100 mg/dl. In contrast, the second study used women with benign breast disease and found results of 70 to 200 mg/dl. These two studies may not be in contradiction; they may represent two different segments of the breast cancer–free group. It is possible that benign breast disease raises the levels of the test to intermediate numerical values.

The proper measure of the disease-free group is the range of normal, which usually includes 95% of the breast cancer–free group. Results here, however, are presented as ranges that include 100% of the individuals; the total range tells nothing about how the results are concentrated. The results may be concentrated heavily between 70 and 100. Without all the data or at least a range of normal, it is difficult to use these studies to compare patients without breast cancer with patients with breast cancer.

Variability Of Those With The Disease

The first study used patients with metastatic breast cancer and found a range of results from 150 to 200 mg/dl. The second study used newly diagnosed breast cancer patients and found a range from 70 to 200. This discrepancy may not reflect error in reporting the data; it may reflect the different groups used. Newly diagnosed breast cancer patients are likely to reflect a wide spectrum of those with the disease. Individuals with early disease as well as metastatic disease are likely to be represented among newly diagnosed patients. Metastatic breast cancer patients, however, may reflect only one end of the spectrum of disease. Thus, the wider range of numerical values found among the newly diagnosed patients may reflect the more representative breast cancer group used in the second study.

Diagnostic Discrimination

The data presented do not allow one to calculate the sensitivity or specificity of the test. No mention is made of the distribution of individual results, so it is not possible to obtain a range of normal or a division between positive and negative tests. Therefore, no conclusions are warranted about the diagnostic utility of the test.

In the first study, the investigators used individuals with a far-advanced disease and individuals who were clearly disease-free. It is not surprising that their test results appeared to separate the groups successfully. In the second study, the investigators included a wider spectrum of the diseased and also included those with benign breast disease. Therefore, it also is not surprising that there was more overlap of numerical values in this second study. The interpretations of the first study as a perfect test and the second study as a worthless test are both incorrect. The truth, which probably lies somewhere in between, requires an assessment of sensitivity and specificity using all the data from a wide spectrum of the diseased and the disease-free groups.

EXERCISE NO. 2: THE CONCEPT OF NORMAL

An investigator attempts to derive the limits of normal for a new test for diabetes in the following way:

1. He locates 1,000 hospital patients admitted for primary conditions other than diabetes.
2. He performs the new test on all 1,000 patients.

3. He plots out the values for the new test, excludes the top 2.5% and the bottom 2.5% and includes the other 95% as the range of normal.

The investigator now takes his new test to the community and performs screening tests on all volunteers. He tells all those who fall within the normal range that they are free of diabetes and tells all those who fall outside the normal range that they have diabetes. One year later he goes back to several individuals whose values fell at the low end of the normal range and retests them. He finds that they are now at the upper end of the normal range, and he assures them that they are free of diabetes.

An obese male patient with results at the high end of the range of normal and a strong family history of diabetes asks for advice on how to avoid developing the disease. The investigator advises him that since he is within the range of normal, he has nothing to worry about.

CRITIQUE: EXERCISE NO. 2

Development Of The Range Of Normal

In developing the range of normal, an investigator should seek to include only individuals who are free of the disease under study. The investigator in the above study concluded that individuals admitted with diagnoses other than diabetes were free of diabetes. Diabetes, however, is a very common condition, and diabetics develop a series of complications that increase their risk of being hospitalized. Therefore, it is likely that a proportion of individuals admitted with other primary diagnoses also had diabetes. The investigator may not have developed his range of normal from diabetes-free patients.

The investigator used the central 95% of the presumably disease-free group's results as the range of normal. This is the usual procedure, but it may not maximize the diagnostic discrimination of the test. By altering the limits of the range of normal, it is sometimes possible to improve the ability of the test to discriminate between those with and those without the disease. It must be remembered, however, that when we change the limits of the range of normal to produce fewer false negative results, we then pay the penalty of producing more false-positive results or vice versa. This penalty may be worth the price, but further data are required before we can know whether this is the case. In any event, these data do not provide adequate means of judging whether this new test helps to discriminate between diabetics and nondiabetics. No external gold standard was used to define who actually had diabetes. All we know is the range of normal for the test.

Applying The Range Of Normal

The distinction between the concept of the range of normal and the concept of pathology has not been maintained. The author has equated outside the range of normal with diabetes and within the range of normal as free of diabetes. No evidence is presented that the new test is of any utility in discriminating diabetics from nondiabetics. It is possible that diabetics fall entirely within the normal range on this test.

Even if this test had been shown to be diagnostically useful in separating those with diabetes from those without diabetes, it is likely that there still would be a few individuals with diabetes within the normal range as well as diabetes-free individuals outside the normal range. By definition, the range of normal excludes 5% of individuals who are free of the disease. Thus the investigator cannot simply apply the test and label individuals as diabetics or nondiabetics.

Changes Within The Range Of Normal

When an individual's results change but remain within the range of normal, it could be a manifestation of pathology. The concept of the range of normal is developed primarily for individuals for whom no previous baseline data are available. When no baseline data for an individual are available, it is necessary to compare an individual's current results with those of supposedly disease free individuals, using the established range of normal. If the same test has been run on the individual previously, this information should be taken into account.

A change within the range of normal may represent a large increase for a given individual; this is especially true if a patient previously had been near the lower limits of the range of normal and then moved to the upper limits. For these individuals, changes within the normal limits may be early manifestations of disease.

Reference Group

The reference group used in the study to develop the range of normal was all hospitalized patients. Their range of normal may have been quite different from those of a younger, ambulatory, and otherwise healthy population. Thus, an error may have been introduced by developing limits of normal from one group and applying it to another group with different characteristics.

Within Normal Limits Versus Desirable

It is possible that all or some of those individuals whose results on the test were within normal limits have numerical values that are higher than desirable. Remember that the range of normal is a reflection of the way things are, not necessarily of how they ideally should be. It is possible that losing weight and thus lowering the test results will prevent future problems. This assumes that the test in fact discriminates between disease and nondiseased, that losing weight will affect the test levels, and that lowered test levels carry a better prognosis. The general point, however, is that results within the range of normal are not necessarily desirable results.

EXERCISE NO. 3: DIAGNOSTIC DISCRIMINATION OF TESTS

The usefulness of a new test for thrombophlebitis is being evaluated. The traditional gold standard for thrombophlebitis has been the venogram to which the new test is being compared. To assess the reproducibility of the new test, it is performed on 100 consecutive patients with positive venograms. The investigators found that 98% of the patients diagnosed as having thrombophlebitis had a positive test result. The investigators then repeated the test on the same group of patients. They again found that it was positive in 98% of the 100 patients. From this they concluded that the new test was 100% reproducible.

Having demonstrated the reproducibility of the new test, the authors proceeded to study its diagnostic discrimination. The authors evaluated the success of the new test as measured against the venogram, the traditional gold standard. They studied 1,000 consecutive patients with unilateral leg pain, 500 of whom had positive venograms and 500 of whom had negative venograms. The investigators classified individuals as positive or negative and presented their data as follows:

NEW TEST	POSITIVE VENOGRAM	NEGATIVE VENOGRAM
Positive	450	100
Negative	50	400
	500	500

The investigators used the accepted definition of sensitivity, that is, sensitivity is the proportion of those with a positive test by the gold standard who have a positive test using the new test. Thus,

$$\text{Sensitivity} = \frac{450}{500} = 0.90 = 90\%$$

They used the accepted definition of specificity, that is, specificity is the proportion of those with a negative test by the gold standard who have a negative test using the new test. Thus,

$$\text{Specificity} = \frac{400}{500} = 0.80 = 80\%$$

They calculated the predictive value of a positive test for their study group. The accepted definition of the predictive value of a positive test is the proportion of those with a positive new test who actually have the condition as measured by the gold standard. Thus,

$$\text{Predictive value of a positive test} = \frac{450}{550} = 0.818 = 81.8\%$$

From these results, the investigators are led to the following conclusions:

1. The new test is completely reproducible.
2. The new test is less sensitive and less specific than the venogram, thus it is an inherently inferior test.
3. When applied to a new group of patients, for instance, a group with bilateral leg pain, a positive new test can be expected to have a predictive value of a positive test equal to 81.8%.

CRITIQUE: EXERCISE NO. 3

If a test is performed several times on the same individuals under the same conditions, the method of assessing reproducibility requires that the results for each individual be nearly identical if the test is 100% reproducible. The authors stated that the total number of positive new tests was identical when the test was repeated. They did not, however, indicate whether the same individuals were positive on repetition of the test as were positive the first time the test was performed. If the same individuals were not positive, the test could not be considered completely reproducible. The authors also failed to indicate whether those who performed and interpreted the repetition of the test knew of the results of the first test.

A gold standard is the generally accepted measure of a disease against which new or unproved tests are compared, but the gold standard traditionally used may not be in fact an ideal measure of the disease it is designed to diagnose. A test used as a gold standard may be considered diagnostic only because tradition or general acceptance have established its usefulness. It is possible, however, for a new test to be a more useful measure of the disease than the accepted gold standard. When comparing the sensitivity and specificity of new tests to that of the gold standard, we must keep in mind that disagreement between the tests may result from a less-than-perfect gold standard instead of the inadequacy of the new test.

When the authors concluded that the new test had lower sensitivity and specificity than the venogram, they were assuming that the venogram was 100% sensitive and 100% specific. When we make this assumption, there is no way for the new test to have a higher sensitivity or specificity than the old test. Unless we can be sure that the venogram is always correct, it is premature to conclude that the new test is a less useful measure of thrombophlebitis. The authors therefore should have limited their conclusions about the sensitivity and specificity of the new test to a comparison to the venogram. If the new test is safer, cheaper, or more convenient than the venogram, it may come to replace the venogram in clinical practice. Clinical experience may eventually demonstrate that it is reliable enough to be used as the gold standard. In the meantime the best the test can do is to match the established gold standard, which by definition has 100% sensitivity and 100% specificity.

The authors have correctly measured the sensitivity, specificity, and predictive value of a positive test for their study group. As they stated, the predictive value of a positive test is the proportion of those with a positive new test who actually have the condition as measured by the gold standard. In this study group the prevalence of thrombophlebitis is 50% (500 with thrombophlebitis, 500 without), and thus the predictive value of the test is 450 per 550 equals 81.8%. The predictive value of a test, however, is different in different groups of patients, depending on the prevalence or pretest probability of the disease in the group being tested. One cannot extrapolate a predictive value derived in one group of patients directly to another group with a different prevalence of the condition. One would expect a group of patients with unilateral leg pain to have a different prevalence of thrombophlebitis from a group of patients with bilateral leg pain.

The predictive values for bilateral leg pain cannot be estimated based solely on the sensitivity and specificity of the test derived from patients with unilateral leg pain. However, if one can also estimate the percentage of those with bilateral leg pain who have thrombophlebitis, then it is possible to estimate the predictive values of a test in patients with bilateral leg pain. Let us assume that the prevalence of thrombophlebitis is much lower among patients with bilateral leg pain. One would then expect that a positive new test would have a much lower predictive value than for a group of patients with unilateral leg pain.

Remember that, clinically, the prevalence is the same as the probability of the disease being present before the test is performed, and the predictive value of a positive test is the probability of the disease being present after obtaining a positive test. Since the probability of thrombophlebitis in a patient who presents with bilateral leg pain is much lower than 50%, the probability of disease even after a positive test would be far below 81.8%.

PART 3

Rating a Rate

CHAPTER 20

Introduction to Rates

When you hear hoof beats, it is more likely to be a horse than a zebra. This clinical pearl stresses the obvious but too often forgotten truth that common diseases occur commonly, and rare diseases occur rarely. When clinicians say that one disease is common and another is rare, they are implying a difference in *rates*.

All clinicians instinctively use a concept of rates. They know that coronary artery disease is much more likely in a middle-aged man than in a teen-aged woman. They know that pancreatic cancer is much more common in an elderly person than in a young person. They know that sickle cell anemia is much more likely to be present in a black person than in a white person.

In our previous discussion of diagnostic tests, we showed that the lower the prevalence rate in a population (i.e., the rarer the disease), the lower the predictive value of a positive test. For a rare disease, then, a positive test is much less likely to indicate disease. Clinicians automatically and perhaps subconsciously employ this concept. They know that a young woman with T-wave changes on an electrocardiogram is unlikely to have coronary artery disease. They know that a young man with persistent abdominal pain is unlikely to have pancreatic cancer. They know that a white person with evidence of joint pain and anemia is unlikely to have sickle cell anemia. The clinician's appreciation of the rates of the disease may be based particularly on clinical experience; however, it is helpful to be able to draw from research articles to gain a more objective and scientific assessment of the rates of disease. This section will aim at assisting the reader to acquire the tools to understand how the rates of disease are scientifically measured and interpreted. Such an understanding helps one to choose the proper diagnostic methods and to interpret the results.

In addition to facilitating individual diagnosis, an appreciation of the rates of illness helps in the assessment of changes that occur over time or as a result of medical intervention. Rates of illness are an important tool for conducting the types of studies that were discussed in *Part 1, Studying a Study.* The ability to identify real changes and true cause and effect relationships is dependent on an understanding of the principles of comparing rates.

It may not be obvious why it is necessary to study the rates of disease. Why not just compare how many times events occur? Let us look at the following example, which illustrates the problems with comparing only the number of events that occur.

A hospital review panel was evaluating the performance of physicians at your hospital. They found that you had five deaths among the 1,000 patients you treated at the hospital last year. The chief of staff had only one death among the 200 patients he treated. The panel decided that since you had five times the number of deaths as the chief of staff, you must have been practicing bad medicine.

You do not have to be prepared to defend yourself by saying, "It might look bad, but I'm really OK!" Instead of looking at the total number of deaths, it is fairer to look at the number of deaths that occurred in relation to the number of deaths that could have occurred. You merely need to point out that your death rate and the chief of staff's were identical: 5 per 1,000 equals 1 per 200. Rates of events have come to your defense. They are worth knowing about!

A probability is a proportion in which the numerator contains the number of times the event occurred and the denominator contains the number of times the event could have occurred. As with all proportions, the numerator is a subset of the denominator. Rates are actually a special type of measure in which the denominator also contains a unit of time.

An important use of rates and proportions in medicine is to characterize the natural history of a disease. Three types of measures are commonly used:

1. Incidence rate: The number of new cases that occur per unit of time
2. Prevalence: The probability of having a disease at a point in time
3. Case-fatality: The probability of dying over a period of time from a disease once it is diagnosed.

Incidence rates are defined as follows:

$$\text{Incidence rate} = \frac{\text{Number of individuals who develop the disease over a period of time}}{\text{Total number of person-years* at risk}}$$

It is often difficult to know how many individuals are at risk of a disease and how long they are at risk. Thus incidence rates are commonly estimated by using the following formula:

$$\text{Incidence rate of a disease} = \frac{\text{Number of individuals who develop the disease over a period of time}}{\substack{\text{Number of individuals in the at-risk} \\ \text{group at mid-point of a time period of} \\ \text{interest} \times \text{the length of the time period}}}$$

If, for instance, one wanted to study the incidence rate at which new cases of duodenal ulcers develop in New York City in 1990, the incidence rate theoretically would be calculated as follows:

$$\substack{\text{Incidence rate of duodenal ulcers} \\ \text{in New York City in 1990}} = \frac{\substack{\text{Number of New York City residents} \\ \text{who developed duodenal ulcers in 1990}}}{\substack{\text{Number of New York City residents at} \\ \text{risk of developing duodenal ulcers} \\ \text{during 1990} \times \text{1 year}}}$$

Since individuals are constantly moving in or out of New York City, it is difficult to know the true number of persons who lived in the city and how long they lived there during 1990. Using a census for New York City on April 1, 1990, one could use this point of time to calculate an approximate incidence rate. The approximate incidence rate of duodenal ulcers in New York City in 1990 then would be calculated as follows:

$$\substack{\text{Incidence rate of duodenal ulcers} \\ \text{in New York City in 1990}} = \frac{\substack{\text{Number of New York City residents} \\ \text{who developed duodenal ulcers in 1990}}}{\substack{\text{Number of New York City residents at} \\ \text{risk of developing duodenal ulcers on} \\ \text{April 1, 1990 (about equal to the number} \\ \text{of New York City residents on} \\ \text{April 1, 1990)} \times \text{1 year}}}$$

The type of rate we have discussed so far is an *incidence* rate, which is related to the risk of developing a disease over a period of time. Risk is the cumulative effect of the incidence rate of disease over a specified

---

* A person-year represents one individual at risk of developing a disease over a period of 1 year.

period of time. We can think of incidence as the speed one is going over a short period of time and risk as the distance one has traveled over a longer period of time, assuming the speed is maintained.* The incidence rate measures the new cases of a particular disease that develop per unit of time, and this may help in examining the cause or etiology of a disease. Risk by estimating the probability of developing a disease over a specified period of time may help if used carefully in prediction of future events. Once a disease occurs, it may be present for a long period of time. Thus, a second type of measurement frequently is used that estimates the probability of *having* a disease at a point in time. Known as *prevalence*, it measures how frequent or prevalent the disease is at any one point in time. The prevalence of disease is very important in diagnosis since it is a starting point for estimating the pretest probability that a disease is present. It provides an estimate of the probability of the presence of disease before evaluating an individual's history, physical examination, or laboratory tests. Thus,

$$\text{Prevalence} = \frac{\text{Number of individuals who have the disease at a point in time}}{\text{Number of individuals who are in the group at the same point in time}}$$

In the previous example, the prevalence of duodenal ulcers on April 1, 1990 in New York City then would be constructed as follows:

$$\text{Prevalence} = \frac{\text{Number of New York City residents with duodenal ulcers on April 1, 1990}}{\text{Number of New York City residents on April 1, 1990}}$$

For most diseases, incidence rate and prevalence are related approximately as follows:

$$\text{Prevalence} = \text{Incidence rate} \times \text{average duration of the disease}$$

In other words, the longer the average duration of the disease, the more individuals will have the disease at any particular time; therefore, the higher the prevalence. Chronic diseases with long duration, such as diabetes, may have a low incidence rate of development of new cases but a high prevalence of the disease at any point in time.

---

* Biostatisticians and epidemiologists distinguish between cumulative incidence and incidence rates. Cumulative incidence contains in the denominator the number of individuals in the population at the beginning of the time period. The cumulative incidence is synonymous with risk.

Acute, short-duration diseases like strep throat may have a high incidence rate of occurrence of new cases but a low prevalence of the disease at any point in time. Thus it is important to appreciate that incidence rates and prevalence measure different phenomena. Incidence rates measure the rate at which a new case of the disease develops per unit of time. Prevalence measures the probability of *having* the disease at a particular time. Failure to appreciate this difference may lead to the type of error illustrated in the following example:

A study of asymptomatic gonorrhea in men was conducted by taking cultures from 1,000 randomly selected asymptomatic men. Ten of these men were found to have gonorrhea. A second study followed a group of men from the same population over a 1-year period. This study found that over 1 year's time only one of these men developed asymptomatic gonorrhea. In comparing the studies, a reviewer concluded that one of them must be wrong since their conclusions were so widely divergent.

This seeming inconsistency is not inconsistent at all if one distinguishes incidence rates from prevalence. The first study of existing cases determined a prevalence; the second assessed the incidence rate. The fact that the prevalence of asymptomatic gonorrhea was much higher than the incidence rate suggests that asymptomatic cases have a long duration. This may be explained by the fact that although symptomatic cases usually receive treatment, asymptomatic cases may remain untreated in the community for a long period of time.

In addition to incidence rate and prevalence, it is necessary to define a third measurement in order to characterize the natural history of a disease. This is known as the *case fatality*.

$$\text{Case fatality*} = \frac{\text{Number of deaths from a disease during a time period}}{\text{Number of individuals diagnosed with the disease at the beginning of the time period}}$$

Case fatality unlike incidence rates is affected by the success of medical interventions designed to cure disease. Since case fatality measures the probability of failing to survive once the disease has developed, case fatality may be helpful in assessing prognosis. Case fatality over a period of time has an important relationship to mortality rates due to a specific disease (i.e., the number of deaths due to a disease per person-year).

---

* Case fatality is a proportion when referring to the probability of eventually dying from a disease. Case fatality is used as a proportion when it is multiplied by incidence rate to produce the mortality rate.

$$\text{Mortality rate} = \text{Incidence rate} \times \text{case fatality}$$

Failure to appreciate this relationship may lead to the type of confusion illustrated in the following situation:

In a study of the rates of duodenal ulcer disease, the authors properly obtained the mortality rates from duodenal ulcers in the United States in 1949 and 1989. In 1949 the yearly mortality rate was 5 per 1,000,000 person-years; in 1989 it was 1 per 1,000,000 person-years. Further study revealed that neither the incidence rate nor the prevalence of duodenal ulcers had changed. The authors could not make sense of these data.

Knowing the relationship between incidence rates and mortality rates, the decline in mortality rate must have been due to a reduced case fatality. This decreased case fatality may reflect progress over 40 years in keeping alive those with duodenal ulcers even if there has been no progress in reducing the incidence rate of new duodenal ulcers.

Incidence rates, prevalence, and case fatality measure the rate of developing new cases of a disease per unit time, the probability of having the disease at a point in time, and the probability of dying from a disease once it is diagnosed. In addition to these basic measures, the medical literature often uses a measurement known as the *proportionate mortality ratio*, which is defined as follows:

$$\text{Proportionate mortality ratio} = \frac{\text{Number of individuals dying from the disease}}{\text{Number of individuals dying from all diseases}}$$

The proportionate mortality ratio measures the probability that a death is due to a particular cause. Proportionate mortality ratios are a useful means of determining which are the most common causes of death. They do not, however, tell us about the probability of death as illustrated in the next scenario.

A well-designed study revealed that trauma was the cause of death in 4% of those over 65-years-old; it caused 25% of the deaths among those under 3-years-old. The authors concluded that those over 65 have a much lower probability of dying from trauma than those under 3-years-old.

The fact that those over 65 have a lower proportionate mortality ratio from trauma does not necessarily mean that the elderly have a lower probability of dying from trauma. Since many more deaths occur among those over 65, even the 4% dying from trauma may represent a mortality rate from trauma that approximates the mortality rate among those under 3-years-old.

Having examined the types of rates and proportions that are most commonly found in the medical literature and having distinguished these measures from ratios, let us turn our attention to the methods for obtaining rates of disease.

CHAPTER 21

Sampling of Rates

Under some circumstances, it is possible to determine every case of a disease in a population. Mortality rates usually can be obtained on entire populations because death certificates are mandatory legal documents. It is often possible therefore to obtain the complete rates of death or mortality rates from a disease for an entire population. For most diseases, however, it is not feasible to count every case of the disease in an entire population, thus the techniques of sampling are very helpful. *Sampling* ideally means that an investigator randomly selects a representative portion of the population, studies this sample, and then tries to extrapolate the results to the entire population that was intended for study.

SAMPLING ERROR

Even when properly performed, the process of sampling is not perfect. To appreciate the process of sampling and the inherent error introduced by sampling, one must understand the basic principle that underlies sampling techniques. This principle states that if many random samples are obtained, rates calculated from data in those samples on the average will be the same as the rate of the original population. In other words, each sample may differ from the original population either by having a higher rate or a lower rate. For example, the following shows an original population rate of 1 per 100,

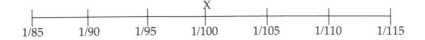

and if the samples were taken from this original population, the rates might look like this:

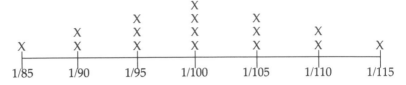

Notice that while some of the rates obtained in particular samples are equal to the rate of the original population, many of them are either higher or lower. Because samples are accurate only on the average, a single sample is said to possess an inherent sampling error. Failure to appreciate the existence of sampling error can lead to the following type of misinterpretation:

A national organization attempted to estimate the prevalence of strep carriers by culturing a random sample of 0.1% of all the school children in the nation. To verify their results, the same organization used a second random sample of 0.1% of the nation's schools and conducted a second survey using an identical protocol. The first survey revealed a prevalence of 15 per 1,000 positive strep cultures; the second survey revealed a prevalence of 10 per 1,000. The authors concluded that the inconsistent results were impossible since they had used the same methodology.

The authors failed to take into account the fact that sampling has an inherent error. This sampling error may be able to explain the differences observed in the two samples. This example merely points out that two identically conducted samples may produce different results on the basis of chance alone. Remember that large numbers of samples, on the average, produce measurements that are identical with the true numerical value for the population, but that any two samples may vary widely from one another and from the true numerical value in the larger population.

SAMPLE SIZE

A second important principle in understanding sampling says that the more individuals who are included in a sample, the more likely a particular sample's rate will closely approximate the rate in the larger population. Thus it is the size of the sample that determines how close the sample rate is likely to be to the rate of the larger population. This is not surprising since when everyone in the population is included in the sample, then the sample's rate is guaranteed to equal the population's rate.

Let us look more closely at this principle. The major factor affecting the size of the sampling error is the size of the sample. The relationship between sample size and precision is not one to one; it is a square root function. With small sample sizes, increasing the size of the sample may greatly increase the precision of the sample's estimate of the population rate. As the sample gets larger, however, diminishing returns set in, and small or moderate increases in sample size may add little to the precision of the estimate. Investigators therefore attempt to balance the need for precision against the financial costs of increasing the sample size. The consequence of using small sample sizes is that the samples may vary widely from one sample to another and from the true numerical value in the larger population. The following example illustrates the need to take into account the effects of sample size on the results of sampling.

An investigator who sampled 0.01% of the nation's death certificates found that the mortality rate from pancreatic cancer was 50 per 100,000 person-years. A second investigator who sampled 1% of the nation's death certificates concluded that the true mortality rate for the nation was 80 per 100,000 person-years. To settle this dispute, the second investigator identified all deaths due to pancreatic cancer in the country. He obtained a rate of 79 per 100,000 person-years. The second investigator concluded that the first investigator had performed his study fraudulently.

The first study used a sample size only one-hundredth as large as the second study; therefore, it is likely that the sampling error of the first study was much larger. The fact that the second large sample turned out to be more accurate is most likely due to its greater precision because of its larger sample size rather than fraud.

RANDOM SAMPLING

Having outlined two important principles of sampling, one further point is left to consider. These two principles rest on the assumption that the sampling has been randomly obtained, meaning that all individuals in the population have an equal probability (or at least a known probability) of being chosen for inclusion in the sample. Unless random sampling is performed, one cannot accurately estimate how close the sample results are to those of the larger population. The need for random sampling is illustrated in the following example:

An investigator from one county hospital estimated that the community rate of myocardial infarction was 150 per 100,000 person-years. An investigator at a private hospital in the same community estimated that the rate was 155 per 100,000 person-years. Since their results were similar, the investigators concluded that the rate of myocardial infarctions in their community must be between 150 and 155 per 100,000 person-years.

Neither of these studies attempted to obtain a random sample of the larger community population. It is possible that myocardial infarction patients either selectively chose these two hospitals or selectively avoided them. If all the area hospitals were included in the sample, the rate of myocardial infarction might have been quite different. The rates in this example were calculated from conveniently available data known as *chunk sampling*. It is the simplest sampling to perform since the investigators merely calculate the rates for an easily available sample. The nonrepresentativeness of a chunk sample, however, means that it cannot be easily or reliably extrapolated to a larger population.*

When obtaining a random sample, investigators will often permit all individuals in the population to have an equal probability of being selected for inclusion in the sample. This is known as a *simple random sample*. Many investigators have found that if they rely exclusively on simple random sampling, they will fail to include enough individuals who possess the characteristics of interest for their study. For instance, if investigators are studying the rates of hypertension in the United States, they may be especially interested in the rates of hypertension for blacks or Orientals. If they merely took a simple random sample of the population, it may not include very many blacks or Orientals. Therefore, investigators could separately sample from blacks, from Orientals, and from the rest of the population. This separate procedure of obtaining random samples from the different subsets or strata of the population is known as *stratified random sampling*. It is permissible and often desirable as long as the sampling within each group is random. There are separate statistical methods for use with stratified samples.

Let us review the principles and requirements for sampling.

1. On the average, samples drawn from a population will have the same rate as in the original population. There is, however, an inherent sampling error introduced by including only a portion of the population.

---

* Occasionally, however, we are forced to make extrapolations from chunk samples. The most common example occurs when we desire to extrapolate research observations to patients seen in the future. Time is one aspect of a population that cannot be randomly sampled.

2. The size of the sampling error is affected by the size of the sample obtained. Increasing the sample size decreases the size of the sampling error, but diminishing returns set in as we increase the size of the sample.

3. The principles of sampling rest on the assumption that samples are randomly obtained. It is permissible to ensure adequate numbers in each category of interest by stratified sampling. However, sampling must be random within each category or stratum. If random sampling is not performed, no method exists of accurately relating the rate obtained in the sample to the true rate of the larger population from which the sample was drawn.

CHAPTER 22

Standardization of Rates

In the previous chapter we outlined the requirements for accurately obtaining rates using random sampling. Here, we will attempt to compare the rates once they are obtained. We will assume that the rates have been properly obtained and illustrate the precautions that must be observed in comparing rates, even those that are measured using proper random sampling techniques.

We will compare rates from samples of two different groups. These groups may be two hospitals, two cities, two countries, two factories, or the same hospital, cities, or factories compared at different points in time. We will compare rates to determine the size of the difference in rates between populations or the extent of change in rates over time. These comparisons are important for rates derived from sampling as well as for rates determined by using an entire population.

When using rates to compare probabilities or risks of disease, it is important to consider whether the populations differ by a factor that is already known to affect the risk of the disease. This consideration is the same as the adjustment for confounding variables discussed previously.

In performing a study, the investigator may know already that factors such as age, sex, or race affect the risk of developing a particular disease. At the same time, the investigator would then adjust for, or "standardize," the rates for these factors. The importance of standardization can be seen in the rates of lung cancer. Since age is a known risk factor for lung cancer, little is gained by discovering that a retirement community has a higher rate of lung cancer than the rest of the community. Likewise, if one factory has a younger work force than a second factory, it is misleading to compare the lung cancer rates in the two factories directly, especially if one wishes to draw conclusions about the safety of working conditions.

To circumvent this problem, rates of disease can be adjusted to take into account the factors that are already known to greatly affect the risks. This process of adjustment of rates is known as *standardization*. Age is the most common factor that requires standardization, but we can adjust for any factor known to have an effect. For instance, using the techniques of standardization to compare the rates of hypertension in two samples to study the importance of differences in the water supply, one might adjust for race since blacks are known to have a higher rate of hypertension.

The principle used in standardizing rates is the same as that used to adjust for the differences in study groups discussed in *Part 1, Studying a Study*. Investigators compare rates among individuals who are similar in age or any other factor that is being adjusted. Before illustrating the method used for adjustment, let us see just how misleading results can occur if standardization is not performed.

The incidence of pancreatic cancer in the United States was compared to the incidence of the same cancer in Mexico. The rate in the United States was found to be three times the rate in Mexico per 100,000 person-years. The authors concluded that Americans are at three times greater risk of pancreatic cancer than Mexicans, assuming that the accuracy of diagnosis were equal in the two countries.

This interpretation of this study is superficially correct; if the data are reliable, the risk of pancreatic cancer is higher in the United States. However, pancreatic cancer is known to occur more often in older persons. It may be that the younger age of the Mexican population accounts for the difference in rate of pancreatic cancer. This may be an important question if we are examining the cause of pancreatic cancer. If the age distribution does not explain these differences, then the investigators may have detected an important, unexpected difference that requires further explanation. Thus authors should standardize their data for age and see if the differences persist.

Standardization of rates is often performed comparing a special sample that is being studied to the general population. In performing this type of standardization we often use what is called the *indirect method*. This method compares the observed number of events such as death in the sample of interest to the number that would have been expected if the study sample had the same age distribution as the general population. When death is the outcome of interest, the indirect method produces a ratio known as the *standardized mortality ratio*.

$$\text{Standardized mortality ratio} = \frac{\text{Observed number of deaths}}{\text{Expected number of deaths}}$$

The standardized mortality ratio is a useful means of comparing a sample from a population of interest to the general population. When interpreting this ratio, however, it is important to remember that a special population under study is often one that is not expected to have the same mortality rate as the general population.

For instance when comparing a group of employed individuals to the general population, it is important to remember that employment often requires that individual be healthy or at least not disabled. The need to take into account this employment effect is illustrated in the next example:

A study of new workers at a chemical plant found a standardized mortality ratio of 1 for all causes of death. The investigator concluded that since the standardized mortality ratio was 1, the chemical plant was free of health risks to the workers.

When interpreting this study it is important to remember that new workers are often healthier than persons in the general population. Thus we would expect them to have a somewhat lower mortality rate than in the general population. This standardized mortality ratio of 1 or 100% thus may fail to reflect risks to these generally healthy workers.

When two groups from a population are under study or when *changes over time* in a population are being assessed, it is desirable to use the direct method of standardization. The direct method works as follows: Suppose investigators wish to compare the rates of bladder cancer in two large industries. The bladder cancer data for the two industries are shown in Table 22-1. Notice that the overall rates for both samples are 200 per 100,000 workers. Also, notice that the rates for each age group are as high or higher in factory A than in factory B. Despite the lower rates for each age group in factory B, it may at first seem surprising that the overall rates are the same. However, looking at the number of individuals in each age group, it becomes apparent that factory A has a much younger work force than factory B. Factory B has 60,000 workers from ages 50 to 70 years; factory A has only 30,000 workers is these age groups. Since bladder cancer is known to increase with age, the younger age of factory A's work force reduces the overall rates in factory A. Thus, it is misleading to look only at the overall rates since factory B's overall rate is increased by its older age structure. This is especially true if we are asking questions about the safety of the factory environment itself.

To avoid this problem, the authors must standardize the rates to adjust for the differences in age and thereby compare the rates more fairly. To accomplish standardization, each sample is subdivided to indicate the number of individuals, the number of cases of the disease, and the incidence rate in each age group. When data are divided into

TABLE 22-1. COMPARISON OF RATES OF BLADDER CANCER

Age	Number of individuals	Number of cases of bladder cancer	Rate of bladder cancer in each age group*
		FACTORY A	
20–30	20,000	0	0 per 100,000
30–40	20,000	10	50 per 100,000
40–50	30,000	20	67 per 100,000
50–60	20,000	80	400 per 100,000
60–70	10,000	90	900 per 100,000
Total	100,000	200	200 per 100,000
		FACTORY B	
20–30	10,000	0	0 per 100,000
30–40	10,000	4	40 per 100,000
40–50	20,000	6	30 per 100,000
50–60	50,000	140	280 per 100,000
60–70	10,000	50	500 per 100,000
Total	100,000	200	200 per 100,000

*The rate is obtained from the number of cases and the number of individuals in the age group. The rates cannot be added down the column.

groups by a characteristic such as age, each division of the data is known as a *strata*. This has been done already and is shown in Table 22-1.

The authors then must attempt to determine how many cases of bladder cancer would have occurred in factory A if the age distribution were the same as in factory B. The steps in this process are as follows:*

1. Starting with the 20 to 30 age group, the authors take the rate of cancer for that group in factory A and multiply this by the number of individuals in the corresponding age group in factory B. This produces the number of cases that would have occurred in factory A if it had the same number of individuals in that age group as factory B.

2. The authors then perform this calculation for each age group and add up the total number of cases from the different age groups. This produces a total number of cases that would have occurred if factory A had the same overall age distribution as factory B.

---

* The method illustrated is not necessarily the only or best method to use for standardization. For statistical purposes, it is common to weight the strata by the inverse of the variance of the estimate in each strata as is done in the Mantel-Haenszel method.

TABLE 22-2. METHOD OF AGE STANDARDIZATION

Age group	Rate of bladder cancer in factory A	Number of individuals in factory B	Number of cases that would occur in factory A if it had the same age distribution as factory B*	Number of cases of bladder cancer that actually occurred in factory B
20–30	0/100,000	10,000	0	0
30–40	50/100,000	10,000	5	4
40–50	67/100,000	20,000	13	6
50–60	400/100,000	50,000	200	140
60–70	900/100,000	10,000	90	50
Totals		100,000	308	200

*This column is calculated by multiplying the previous two columns.

3. The authors now have standardized the rates for age and can directly compare the number of cases that occurred in factory B with the number of cases that would have occurred in factory A if factory A had the same age distribution as factory B. The authors have now age-adjusted factory A to factory B's age distribution."

Let us apply these procedures to the bladder cancer data as shown in Table 22-2.

Three hundred and eight cases of bladder cancer would have occurred in factory A if the age distribution were the same as factory B, but only 200 actually did occur in factory B. These figures are better measures for comparing the risk to the workers of developing bladder cancer in each factory than are the unadjusted frequencies. The adjusted numbers accentuate the fact that despite the equality of the overall rates, factory A has a rate as high or higher in each age group. Therefore, in order to make fair comparisons between populations which differ by age and where age is known to affect the risk of disease, it is necessary to age-standardize the samples. If additional factors are also known to affect the rates, the same process can be applied to standardize or adjust for these factors.

Standardization produces summary measures of large quantities of data, thus it is tempting to standardize data whenever one is comparing two groups.

---

* It is also possible to age-adjust the opposite way, thus age-adjusting factory B to factory A's age distribution. The general conclusion would be the same; however, the estimates would be different.

TABLE 22-3. COMPARISON OF MORTALITY RATES FROM CYSTIC FIBROSIS, 1969 AND 1989

Age (yr)	Mortality rate	Population	Total No. of deaths
	1969		
0–10	5/100,000	1,000,000	50
10–20	10/100,000	1,000,000	100
20–40	1/100,000	2,000,000	20
		4,000,000	170
	1989		
0–10	3/100,000	1,000,000	30
10–20	6/100,000	1,000,000	60
20–40	4/100,000	2,000,000	80
		4,000,000	170

Notice, however, that in performing standardization, the calculations give special emphasis or "weight" to the largest subgroups. Thus if there has been a substantial change in only one subgroup, especially a small subgroup, this effort can easily be lost in the process of standardization. In addition progress may be made by delaying death. When death from a particular cause is moved from a younger to an older age group, this effect may be lost in the process of standardization as illustrated in the following study:

A study of the mortality rates due to cystic fibrosis was conducted to determine whether progress in therapy for children was reflected in the mortality rates of a large state with a stable population distribution. A comparison of data from 1969 and 1989 is shown in Table 22-3.

Notice in this example that the mortality rate from cystic fibrosis for those 0 to 10 and 10 to 20 years of age has fallen between 1969 and 1989. However, the mortality rate from cystic fibrosis among 20- to 40-year-olds has increased from 1969 to 1989. This increase is balanced by the decrease among younger individuals so that the overall crude mortality rates in both years were 170 per 4,000,000 or 4.25 per 100,000 person-years. It is tempting to try to standardize these rates and obtain an adjusted measure of mortality rate. However, if we were to standardize by applying the 1989 age distribution to the 1969 mortality rates (or vice versa), the results after adjustment would be no different from the overall crude rates before adjustment. This occurs because the 1969 and 1989 populations have the same age distribution.

Unfortunately standardization does not help us to see what is happening here. The unadjusted or crude and the standardized rates both obscure the fact that a substantial decrease in mortality rates has occurred among those 0 to 10 and 10- to 20-years-olds. To recognize that this change has occurred, it is necessary to look directly at the actual data for each age group.*

It is important to appreciate that both crude and age-adjusted rates may fail to reveal differences or changes that occur in only one or a few age groups. Changes in one age group are especially likely to be missed when other age groups are changing in opposite directions.

One situation where these opposing changes frequently occur is when death is being delayed until an older age but cure does not occur. This principle is important to understand in order to appreciate the error in the following study:

An investigator studied a new treatment for breast cancer that prolonged the survival of stage 2 breast cancer by an average of 5 years. He confidently predicted that if his new treatment was widely applied, the overall age-adjusted mortality rate from breast cancer would dramatically fall over the next 20 years.

This investigator failed to recognize that when life is prolonged but death is moved to later years, this does not necessarily result in progressively improving overall age-adjusted mortality rates. Despite the success of this new breast cancer therapy, the authors are not claiming cure. When life is prolonged, individuals may die of the disease at an older age. When this occurs, the breast cancer mortality rates in the younger age groups may fall whereas the breast cancer mortality rates in the older age groups may rise. Thus the overall age-adjusted mortality rates may not reveal the progress that has been made.

---

* In addition it is possible to apply statistical methods that produce measurements known as *life-expectancy*. Life expectancy takes into account the impact of the increased years of life lived even in the absence of a cure. Life expectancy is obtained from cross-sectional life tables that assess the hypothetical probability of survival for the average individual who reaches a particular age. Assuming stable mortality experience, life expectancy is based on the mortality experience of a particular population, such as the U.S. population, in a particular calendar year.

CHAPTER 23

Sources of Differences in Rates

In this chapter, let us assume that it has been established that two groups have different rates. These differences between rates may represent differences between two groups or differences over time in the same group.

ARTIFACTUAL DIFFERENCES OR CHANGES

The differences in rates may be the result of real changes in the natural history of the disease itself or they may reflect changes or differences in the method by which the disease under consideration is assessed. *Artifactual differences* imply that, despite the fact that a difference exists, the difference is not a reflection of changes in the disease but merely in the way the disease is measured, sought, or defined.

Artifactual changes result from three sources:

1. Changes in the *ability* to recognize the disease. These represent changes in the measurement of the disease.
2. Changes in the *efforts* to recognize disease. These may represent efforts to recognize the disease at an earlier stage, changes in reporting requirements or new incentives to search for the disease.
3. Changes in the *definition* of the disease. These represent changes in the terminology used to define the disease.

The following example illustrates the first type of artifactual change, the effect of a change in the ability to recognize a disease:

Because of a recent increase in interest, a study of the prevalence of mitral valve prolapse was performed. A complete survey of the charts at a major university cardiac clinic found that in 1969 only 1 per 1,000 patients had a diagnosis of mitral valve prolapse, whereas in 1989, 80 per 1,000 had mitral valve prolapse included in their diagnosis. The authors concluded that the condition was increasing at an astounding rate.

Between 1969 and 1989 the use of echocardiography greatly increased the ability to document mitral valve prolapse. In addition, the growing recognition of the frequency of this condition led to a much better understanding of how to recognize it by physical examination. It is not surprising then that a much larger proportion of cardiac clinic patients were known to have mitral valve prolapse in 1989 compared to 1969. It is possible that if an equal understanding and equal technology were available in 1969, the rates would have been nearly identical. This example demonstrates that artifactual changes may explain large differences in the rates of disease even when a complete review of all cases is used to calculate the prevalence of disease.

Changes in the efforts to recognize disease may occur when physicians attempt to diagnose disease at an earlier stage. If a screening program is introduced to diagnose a disease at a stage when no symptoms exist, then individuals are likely to be diagnosed sooner. The efforts at earlier diagnosis produce a greater "lead time" in diagnosis compared to the previous method. If the available treatment is more successful when applied earlier, then this may result in an improved outlook or prognosis. If, however, no adequate treatment exists or early treatment makes no difference, then we may be merely increasing the interval between diagnosis and death. This may produce an artifactual difference if the rate of death is measured in the immediate time period after diagnosis. An example of this lead-time bias is illustrated in the following example:

Prior to the introduction of an x-ray screening program for lung cancer, the 6-month case fatality was 80 per 100 diagnosed cases. After the introduction of the screening program, the 6-month case fatality was 20 per 100 diagnosed cases. The authors concluded that the screening program had drastically lowered the case fatality from lung cancer and thus had proved its importance.

The screening program probably diagnosed cases of lung cancer at an asymptomatic stage versus the previous diagnosis that occurred after symptoms were present. Evidence suggests the long-term prognosis of lung cancer is not altered by x-ray screening. X-ray screening probably merely alters the lead time between diagnosis and death, producing a lead-time bias. Thus the observed changes are probably artifactual due to the earlier recognition of the disease.

The following example illustrates how the meaning of terminology may change over time and thus produce an artifactual change in the rate of events:

The incidence rate of acquired immunodeficiency syndrome (AIDS) increased every year between 1981 and 1986. In 1987 there was a sudden 50% increase in the reported rate. One investigator interpreted this sudden increase as a sign that the epidemic had suddenly entered a new phase.

In 1987 there was a change in the Centers for Disease Control's definition of AIDS, which meant that more individuals with human immunodeficiency virus (HIV) infection fell within the definition of AIDS. When sudden changes in the incidence rates of a disease occur, one must suspect artifactual changes such as changes in the definition of a disease. Here one suspects that an artifactual change was superimposed on a real change, complicating the interpretation of the data.

REAL CHANGES

Artifactual changes in rates imply that the true incidence rate prevalence or case fatality has not been altered even though superficially a change appears to have occurred. Real changes, however, imply that the incidence rates, prevalence, or case fatality have actually changed. We first must ask whether any of the sources of artifactual differences are operating. If they are not operating or are not large enough to explain the differences, one can assume that real differences or changes exist. Having established that real differences or changes have occurred, we need to ask why these changes occur. Do they reflect a change in incidence rates, prevalence, case fatality, or a combination of these measurements?

The first step in understanding the meaning of a real change in rates is to understand where in the natural history of the disease a change occurred. Then we can better appreciate the effects of the primary changes on the other rates of disease, for instance in the following cases:

1. The case fatality for Hodgkin's disease has dramatically decreased in recent years. Individuals are considered to have the disease until they demonstrate evidence of cure in long-term follow-up. Thus the prevalence of Hodgkin's disease has increased. The incidence rates have remained stable; therefore, the mortality rates, which reflect the incidence rates times the case fatality, have fallen.

2. Lung cancer incidence rates have increased dramatically over recent decades. The case fatality, however, has remained very low

with most patients dying within months of diagnoses. Thus the mortality rates have also increased dramatically. Because of the short duration of the disease, the prevalence has always been low; however, with the increased incidence rate of disease, it has risen slightly.

We might diagram these results as follows:

	MORTALITY RATES	CASE FATALITY	INCIDENCE RATES	PREVALENCE
Hodgkin's disease	↓	↓↓↓	→	↑↑
Lung cancer	↑↑	→	↑↑	↑

These confusing patterns make sense when one recognizes that the primary change in Hodgkin's disease has been the decreased case fatality whereas the primary change in lung cancer has been the increased incidence rate.

In addition to understanding the source of the differences or changes in rates, it is often tempting to use past changes in rates to predict future rates.

Predicting future rates from current rates or recent changes in rates, or both, is an extremely difficult job. A recent change in rates may have any of the following meanings: (1) These changes may herald future changes in the same direction; (2) they may reflect predictable cycles or epidemics; or (3) they may be the result of unpredictable chance fluctuations representing an unusual frequency of events. Before concluding that observed changes in rates are likely to continue, one must consider the possibility either of cyclical or chance fluctuations. If a natural cycle occurs in the frequency of the disease, the rate from year to year may look like Figure 23-1.

If investigators should note the increase that occurred between 1981 and 1984, they may attempt to measure the changes between 1985 and 1987 and would again find an increase. It is important, however, that investigators realize that this real change between 1981 and 1987 may be part of the natural cycle of disease. It does not necessarily imply that a further increase can be expected in 1988, 1990, or 1995.

As opposed to this predictable cycle of disease, there may be an unpredictable, chance variation in the rate of disease from year to year (Fig. 23-2). In this situation, if investigators pick a year where the rate was higher and compare it to the next year, where by chance alone the rate was lower, they may believe they are documenting important changes when, in fact, they are merely discovering the statistical principle of *regression to the mean*. Statistical regression to the mean or return to the average states that unusual values are by definition rare

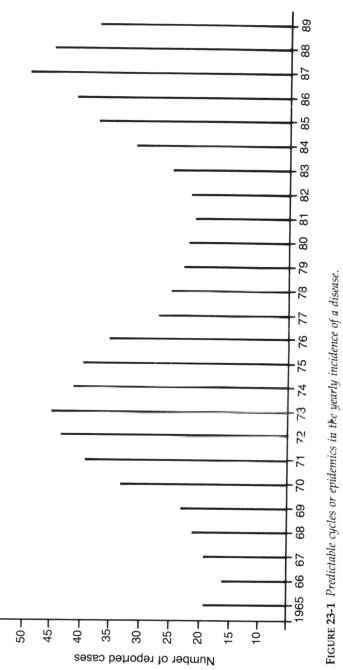

FIGURE 23-1 *Predictable cycles or epidemics in the yearly incidence of a disease.*

211

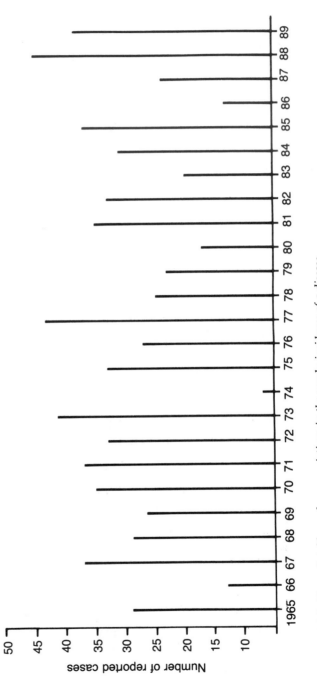

FIGURE 23-2 *Unpredictable or chance variations in the yearly incidence of a disease.*

events, and the odds are against a repetition of a rare event twice in a row. In fact, by chance alone, the next measurement is likely to be nearer the average value.

Subsequent values may be more extreme than an observed value because of chance fluctuation of events or because of forces that react to the unusual rate and move it into line or back toward the average or mean. For instance, if one were studying how much an individual eats per meal, it is likely that the meal following an indulgence would be smaller than usual. Let us see how this principle may operate in a study of rates that produced real differences, but differences that need to be carefully interpreted.

After a tragic accident that killed several men in a factory, an accident prevention program was initiated. Investigators found that the incidence rate of accidents at the time of the tragedy was unusually high—10 per 1,000 workdays. The rate fell to 2 per 1,000 workdays when the program was established. The investigators concluded that the accident prevention program was an enormous success.

The investigators have shown that a real change took place. They have not, however, shown that it was the accident prevention program that caused the change. It is possible that the 10 per 1,000 rate was unusually high and by chance alone returned to a more usual rate of 2 per 1,000. Even more likely, the fatal accident may have frightened the workers into taking more safety precautions, producing what might be called a *psychological regression* to the mean. The authors started with an unusually high accident rate, and then a tragedy occurred that could have forced the rate back toward the mean or average. The authors documented a true change but one that may be explained by regression to the mean rather than a long-lasting change. It is premature to conclude that the accident prevention program would help other groups or even this group if it were done at another time. Thus, the principle of regression to the mean may be the source of real changes in rates, but this source of real changes may have limited importance and may imply that observed changes are not guaranteed to continue.

It is common for an investigation to be initiated because of a suspicion that the rates of disease are increasing. Thus it is important to recognize the phenomenon of regression to the mean because it may start operating whenever short-term changes in rates are observed.

Another source of real differences that affect prediction of future events is known as the *cohort effect*. A *cohort* is a group of individuals who share a common experience or exposure. If one or several cohorts in a population have undergone an exposure or experience that makes them particularly susceptible to disease, then the possibility of a cohort effect exists. The rates for a particular age group, which includes the susceptible cohort, may be temporarily increased. This temporary increase is known as the cohort effect. When a cohort effect is present, one can expect the rates for this particular age group to fall again as time passes and the susceptible cohort passes beyond this particular age group. The importance of appreciating the cohort effect is illustrated in the following example:

An investigator was studying the incidence rate of thyroid cancer. Concern existed that past pediatric head and neck radiation frequently used before 1950 was a contributor to thyroid cancers. Using proper methods, the authors found that the incidence rate of thyroid cancer among the 20- to 30-year age group in 1950 was 50 per 100,000 person-years; in 1960 it was 100 per 100,000 person-years; and in 1970 it was 150 per 100,000 person-years. The authors concluded that by 1980, the rates would pass the 200 per 100,000 person-years mark. The authors were surprised to find that the incidence rate in 1980 was less than 150 per 100,000 person-years and continued to decline during the 1980s.

The authors have established that real changes were occurring in the incidence rates of thyroid cancer in the 20- to 30-year age group. The source of these changes may be a cohort effect. The cohort of individuals who were radiated before 1950 carried an increased risk of thyroid cancer that did not necessarily affect those individuals who were born after 1950. By 1980, all individuals in the 20- and 30-year age group would have been born after 1950. Thus, it is not surprising to observe a decline in the incidence rate of thyroid cancer in 20- to 30-year-olds rather than a continued rise. The concept of a cohort effect not only helps predict the expected future rates, it also helps to support the theory that past radiation increased the risk of thyroid cancer.

Regression to the mean and the cohort effect are two reasons why it is dangerous to predict future rates of disease by direct extrapolation from recent changes in rates. In addition to the comparison of rates in samples from the same group over time, it is also possible to use rates to examine differences between samples from different groups. Comparison of rates in groups is often done to generate hypotheses that can then be tested by the types of investigations we discussed in *Part 1, Studying a Study*. Investigators for instance might note differences in rates of coronary artery disease mortality among Alaskan Eskimos and Alaskan whites. From what they know about the diet of Alaskan Eskimos, they might hypothesize an association between fish consumption and reduced coronary artery mortality.

By comparing the rates of disease and adjusting for known risk factors, it is possible to establish that a factor is increased in one group and a disease is also increased in the same group. This allows us to establish *group associations*. A group association implies that in a particular group, the factor and the disease are both present with increased prevalence. Notice a group association does not necessarily imply that those individuals with the factor are the same individuals as those with the disease.

Establishing the existence of a group association may lay the groundwork for subsequent studies that establish an association at the individual level and eventually a cause and effect relationship such as in the case of cholesterol and coronary artery disease.

When using group data, the investigators frequently have little information about the individuals who make up the group. Thus when comparing rates to develop a hypothesis for further study, investigators must be careful not to imply an association among individuals when only a group association has been established. This type of error, known as an *ecological fallacy*, is illustrated in the following example:

A study demonstrated that the rate of drowning in Florida is four times that in Illinois. The study data also demonstrated that in Florida, ice cream is consumed at a rate four times that of Illinois. The authors concluded that eating ice cream is associated with drowning.

To establish an association, the authors must first demonstrate that those who eat more ice cream are the ones who are more likely to drown. Relying on group figures alone does not provide any information about the existence of an association at the individual level. It may not be those who eat ice cream who drown. The greater consumption of ice cream may merely reflect the confounding variable known as warm weather, which increases ice cream consumption and drowning. These authors committed an ecological fallacy. The establishment of an association between eating ice cream and drowning requires a demonstration that the relationship holds on an individual level.

When faced with differences in rates between groups or changes over time in the same group, the first step is to establish whether the difference or changes are artifactual or real. If it is not likely that the differences or changes are due to the way the disease is measured, sought, or defined, then one can consider that the changes or differences are real. The source of the differences or changes is then sought in the incidence rate, prevalence, or case fatality. Changes or differences in rates are often used to predict future changes and to form hypotheses about the etiology of disease to be used as the basis for studies of individuals. When predicting future rates, regression to the mean and the cohort effect must be taken into account. When using rates in groups to develop hypotheses, it must be recognized that the use of group rates establishes group and not individual association. Failure to appreciate the distinction between group and individual association may lead to an ecological fallacy.

CHAPTER 24

Summary: Rating a Rate

Let us review the steps required for development, comparison, and interpretation of rates of disease.

SELECTION OF RATES

Incidence rates are important clinical measures since they measure the rate at which new cases of diseases develop. Risk is the cumulative effect of the incidence rate over a specified period of time. Prevalence helps in diagnosis by approximating the probability of having a disease at a particular point in time. Case fatality measures the probability of dying due to a disease once the disease is diagnosed. The prevalence is approximately equal to the incidence rate times the average duration of the disease. In a stable population, the mortality rate equals the incidence rate times the case fatality.

SAMPLING OF RATES

Rates may be derived by using the entire larger population. More frequently, rates are estimated using only samples from the larger population. The sample rates, on the average, are the same as the larger population, but any one sample may reflect an inherent sampling error. The larger size of the sample, the smaller the sampling error will be. However, diminishing returns set in as the size of the samples increase and the investigators must weigh accuracy against cost. The ability to estimate the rate of disease in a population from a sample requires random sampling from the population. It is possible to stratify the sample to ensure great enough numbers in each category, but sampling must be random within each category.

STANDARDIZATION OF RATES

Whether obtained by inclusion of the entire population or by sampling, one is interested in comparing rates to estimate the differences between groups or changes over time. When comparing rates, a fair comparison often requires that the rates be adjusted for factors known to affect the rate of disease, which are different in the two samples. Demographic factors such as age, sex, and race are frequently adjusted or standardized to look for other factors that produce the differences or changes in rates. Indirect standardization can produce a standardized mortality ratio that compares the rate in a particular study group to that expected from the rate in another group, often the general population. The direct method of standardization allows one to compare groups directly after standardizing or adjusting for a characteristic that differs in the two groups.

SOURCES OF CHANGES OR DIFFERENCES

The meaning of the differences is assessed by examining the differences to determine whether they are artifactual or real. Changes in ability to recognize the disease, efforts to recognize the disease, or definition of the disease may produce artifactual changes or differences that are not due to changes or differences in the disease itself.

If artifactual differences or changes are not great enough to explain the observed differences or changes, then a real difference or change is assumed to be present. Real changes may result from changes in the incidence rate, the prevalence, or the case fatality. These real changes may herald further changes in the same direction, or they may be followed by declining rates as an epidemic subsides. Alternatively they may reflect chance fluxuations in the rates of disease. When using changes in rates to predict future rates, it is important to recognize a phenomenon known as *regression to the mean*. This effect often occurs when the original rate used for comparison is unusual. This unusual rate may set forces in motion that help bring the future rates back toward or even below the average. Biostatisticians use the term *regression to the mean* to indicate that by chance alone after the occurrence of an unusual value, subsequent measurements are likely to be closer to the mean or average value.

Another type of real change in rates is known as the *cohort effect*. The cohort effect, by isolating the changes to one segment of the population, helps to predict future rates better than mere extrapolation from the observed changes. The study of the sources of real changes in rates helps one to better understand their causes as well as their consequences for subsequent years.

When using differences in rates to develop hypotheses for conducting studies on individuals, it must be recognized that group associations are established using rates. Ecological fallacies are possible when group associations are not reflected at the individual level.

QUESTIONS TO ASK IN RATING A RATE

The following set of questions to ask in rating a rate is designed to review the areas covered and to provide an outline for use in critiquing a flaw-catching exercise or a real investigation of rates. It is divided into selecting a rate, sampling of rates, standardization of rates, and sources of changes or differences in rates.

1. Selection of rates
   a. Were the distinctions between rates, proportions, and ratios recognized?
   b. Did the authors distinguish between an incidence rate, prevalence and case fatality?
2. Sampling of rates
   a. Was the entire population of interest included in the study, or were samples used?
   b. If samples were used, did the authors appreciate the inherent sampling error?
   c. If samples were used, was the sampling technique random or representative, or was bias introduced by the method of sampling?
   d. If samples were used, were the sizes of the samples adequate, or was it likely that a large variation was introduced by the small sample size?
3. Standardization of rates
   a. Was standardization necessary when comparing the rates of occurrence of an event in two different samples?
   b. If standardization was necessary, were the rates standardized for factors that are known to affect outcome so that the rates could be fairly compared?

4. Sources of changes or differences in rates
   a. Were the observed changes or differences in rates artifactual due to changes in the ability to recognize the disease, efforts to recognize the disease, or changes in the definition of the disease?
   b. Were real differences or changes due to changes or differences in the incidence rate, prevalence, or case fatality?
   c. Do the changes or differences in rates predict future changes in the same direction, or will future rates be affected by the phenomenon of regression to the mean or a cohort effect?
   d. When using differences in rates to develop hypotheses for further study, was the distinction between group association and association at the individual level maintained?

CHAPTER 25

Flaw-Catching Exercises: Rating a Rate

The following flaw-catching exercises are designed to give you practice in applying the principles of rating a rate to simulated research
articles. The exercises include a variety of errors that have been illustrated in the hypothetical examples. Read each exercise. Then write a
critique pointing out the types of errors committed by the investigators. A sample critique is provided for each exercise.

EXERCISE NO. 1:
CHANGES IN CANCER: WHAT IS PROGRESS?

A study of progress in cancer in the United States compared the rates
in 1969 to the rates in 1989 to assess changes. Data on incidence rates
and mortality rates were collected. Incidence data were obtained from
an intensive search of hospital records on a random sample of 1% of
the nation's hospitals. Data on mortality were obtained from a complete review of all the death certificates in the nation. Case fatality was
derived from the formula for long-term changes, which says that

Mortality rates = incidence rates × case fatality.

The data from these studies is summarized in Table 25–1.
   In addition the researchers reviewed controlled clinical trials on
cancers that caused 50% of the deaths among those 20 years and
older. They found that data from those trials showed an increase in
median survival of 3 years when applying new therapies developed
since 1969.

TABLE 25-1. CHANGES IN CANCER RATES FROM 1969 TO 1989

Age	Incidence Rate	Case fatality	Mortality Rate
0–19	No change	20% decrease	20% decrease
20–65	1% increase	1% decrease	No change
65–	15% increase	10% decrease	5% increase

Finally the researchers calculated the *proportionate mortality ratio* based on a review of the cause of death from all death certificates. They found that the proportionate mortality ratio for cancer overall had increased from 22 to 24%.

The researchers confessed complete confusion saying that it was possible to argue:

1. There has been substantial progress based on the decreased mortality rates for those under 20, the decreased case fatality for all age groups, and the increased survival in controlled clinical trials among those 20 and over.
2. The situation is getting worse based on the increased incidence rates among those over 20 and the increased age-adjusted incidence rate. The increased mortality rates among those over 65 and the increased proportionate mortality rates also support a worsening of the situation.
3. No change has occurred based on the age-adjusted overall mortality rates.

The investigators throw up their hands and ask you the readers to explain how the data could support such inconsistent results.

CRITIQUE: EXERCISE NO. 1

These rates are all compatible. They reflect different ways to look at and different ways to argue about rates. Incidence rates reflect the rate at which new cases of the disease develop over a period of time. Case fatality reflects the probability of dying over a period of time if the disease develops. Thus incidence rates and case fatality measure two very different phenomena. Incidence rates primarily reflect the underlying causes of disease. They may be artifactually changed by medical interventions that alter the effort to detect disease, the ability to detect disease, or the definition of disease. Primary prevention efforts such as cigarette cessation may alter the underlying incidence. In general, however, incidence rates do not reflect the usual therapeutic efforts that go on as part of medical care. Case fatality on the other hand is a measure of the success of medical therapy in its effort to cure disease.

Mortality rates over a long period of time are related to incidence and case fatality as follows:

$$\text{Mortality rates} = \text{incidence rates} \times \text{case-fatality}$$

Thus if the mortality rate and the incidence rate are known and stable, the case fatality can be approximated as follows:

$$\text{Case-fatality} = \frac{\text{Mortality rate}}{\text{Incidence rate}}$$

Therefore the first table correctly used the relationship between incidence rate, and mortality rate, and case fatality.

When a medical intervention successfully prolongs life but does not cure a disease, this intervention has no effect on the overall or long-term case fatality. Thus the 3-year increased median survival among those with major cancers is compatible with the more modest decrease in case fatality observed in the overall age-adjusted data. Life-expectancy measures are needed to take into account the prolongation of life in the absence of cure.

The increased proportionate mortality ratio tells us very little about the progress in cancers over those years. It does suggest, however, that mortality due to other diseases is becoming less frequent compared with cancers. Proportionate mortality ratios are useful measures of the relative importance of various causes of death. The increase in the proportionate mortality ratio suggests that deaths from cancer are becoming more common relative to deaths from other causes.

This exercise demonstrates how it is possible to argue for quite different conclusions from the same data. The argument presented by the researcher reflects different concepts about what is meant by progress. Is progress a reduced incidence rate for new disease? Is progress an increased cure rate for diagnosed disease? Or, is progress a prolongation of life for those with disease?

EXERCISE NO. 2: TUBERCULOSIS

An international group of tuberculosis (TB) experts decided to compare the mortality rate from TB in the United States with that of India to determine if any lessons could be learned. They knew that TB was quite common in the United States before 1950, but that it had declined substantially. They also knew that most individuals who are infected are able to control but not eliminate the infection totally.

Using a carefully designed large random sample technique, the investigators found that the mortality rate due to TB in 1985 was 200 per 100,000 person-years in India versus 20 per 100,000 person-years in the United States. They also found that the mortality rate for individuals in the 65- to 80-year-old age group was 200 per 100,000 person-years in India and 200 per 100,000 person-years in the United States.

Since the investigators knew that India had a much younger population than did the United States and that age affects the risk of TB, they tried to age-standardize the rates. They applied the rates for each age group from the U.S. population to the number of person-years in that age group in India. After direct age adjustment they found that 200 deaths occurred per 100,000 person-years due to TB in India in 1985. They found that there would have been 10 deaths per 100,000 person-years in the United States if there had been the same age distribution in the United States as in India. Finally they calculated the proportional mortality ratio for TB in the two countries. In India they found that TB has a proportionate mortality ratio of 1.5% versus 1% in the United States.

The authors drew the following conclusions:

1. The large difference in mortality rates between India and the United States may have been due to chance.

2. The mortality rate in the United States for the 65- to 80-year-old age group is much higher than the average U.S. rate. Thus as the average age of the U.S. population gets older, TB will become more of a problem.

3. In comparing the unstandardized rates, it appeared that India had 10 times the U.S. rate of TB. Once standardization was completed, it showed that India had 20 times as much TB. Some mistake must have been made since rate standardization should not make the differences in rates look larger than prestandardized rates. Thus contrasting the overall rates was the fairest means of comparison.

4. The proportionate mortality ratios are the fairest way to compare the probability of death from TB. Thus the probability of death from TB was 1.5 times higher in India as compared to the United States.

CRITIQUE: EXERCISE NO. 2

Selection Of Rates

Let us evaluate one by one the conclusions reached by the "experts."

1. It is very unlikely that the differences between the United States and India are due only to chance because of their wide separation and large sample size. However, before concluding that these differences are real, we must consider whether artifactual differences either in effort or in ability to recognize TB occur between the two countries and whether these factors could explain the differences found. If we assume that India—with its enormous health problems—is less able than the United States to recognize TB as the cause of death, this fact would actually increase the already large differences found. Thus, artifactual differences in the effort or ability to recognize deaths from TB are not likely to explain or eliminate the differences found.

2. The authors have noted that the rates among the 65- to 80-year-old age group are identical in the United States and in India. This suggests that the United States experiences a mortality rate among the elderly that is much higher than among the rest of the U.S. population, which may be due to some permanent susceptibility among the U.S. elderly. On the other hand, it may reflect a cohort effect. Remember, a cohort effect is a unique, temporary susceptibility among one group or co- hort due to a special past experience. Historically, we know that TB was a much more common disease in the United States prior to 1950. In addition, we know that individuals who have been previously infected frequently control the infection but often do not eliminate it totally. These individuals have the possibility of subsequently devel- oping active disease, especially when they become elderly. Thus, it is possible that the high rate among the U.S. elderly is related to their experience in an era when active TB was quite frequent. If the cohort effect explains the high TB rate among the U.S. elderly, then it is not likely that the high U.S. rate among those 65- to 80-years-old will continue to increase as the proportion of elderly in the U.S. popula- tion increases. The rates for this age group may actually fall as less susceptible cohorts, those who were not previously exposed to TB, advance into this age group.

In India, on the other hand, the rate for the 65- to 80-year-old age group is the same as the general Indian population. Thus, in India, there is no reason to believe that a cohort effect is operating. The rates for all age groups may be uniformly high, and the elderly do not necessarily share a unique susceptibility. This implies that if the Indian population experiences an increase in the proportion of elderly, they may not experience much change in the mortality rate from TB.

3. The investigators correctly concluded that rate standardization for age was an important procedure if the rates were to be fairly compared. Standardization is important since the populations have a markedly different age distribution, and age is related to the risk of dying from TB. The Indian population is generally younger than the U. S. population. Deaths from TB are concentrated among the old and the very young, thus age standardization is necessary if a fair comparison is to be achieved. The procedure for age standardization was correctly performed. By applying the rates for each age group in the U.S. population to the number of individuals in that age group in the Indian population, the investigators were asking how many deaths would have occurred in the U. S. population if there were the same number of individuals in each age group as in India. This number can then be compared directly to the number of deaths that actually occurred in India. Standardization may make the differences appear smaller or larger. There is no reason to believe that standardization will make big differences look smaller. As illustrated in the factory example during the discussion of standardization (Chap. 22), age adjustment may even reveal an important difference where none was apparent in the overall rates.

4. The proportionate mortality ratio reflects the number of individuals who die from a disease divided from the number who die from all diseases. Since the overall mortality rates are substantially higher in India than in the United States, the denominator of the proportionate mortality ratio for India will be substantially higher. Thus when calculating the proportionate mortality ratio for India, we divide a larger numerator by a larger denominator. Therefore, it is not surprising that we come up with a proportionate mortality ratio for India that is only modestly higher than the proportionate mortality ratio for the United States. The proportionate mortality ratio should not be looked on as a measure of probability of death but rather as a measure of the relative importance of a disease in a particular population.

PART 4

Selecting a Statistic

CHAPTER 26

Basic Principles

Statistics have three purposes in medical research: (1) to summarize great numbers of measurements with a manageable few, (2) to make estimates and inferences from samples obtained from large populations, taking into account the influence of chance, and (3) to adjust for the influence of confounding variables on those estimates and inferences. It is our goal, in *Selecting a Statistic* to provide some insight as to how statistics can be used to serve these purposes. We do not assume that we can, in these few pages, substitute for the involvement of a statistician in the planning, execution, and interpretation phases of most medical research projects; instead, we hope to provide the tools necessary to appreciate the "statistical methods" section for readers of the research literature so that the analysis, interpretation and, extrapolation of research results can be more fully understood.

To use statistics in medical research, we must first choose an appropriate statistical method. Next, research measurements must be manipulated as prescribed by the chosen method. Finally, the results of those manipulations must be correctly interpreted. The first and last of those tasks are intimately related and are the subject of *Part 4, Selecting a Statistic*. We will not, however, make an attempt to discuss the actual data manipulations necessary to generate statistics. Certainly, a richer understanding of statistical methods requires study of those manipulations, but, in our opinion, that level of understanding is not compulsory to be able to evaluate why a particular method is selected and how we can interpret the results of its application.

Let us begin by taking a look at how we approach the first and second of the purposes of statistics. The third purpose of statistics, to adjust for the effect of confounding variables, is accomplished by multivariable analysis. It is addressed in Chapter 29.

SUMMARIZING MEASUREMENTS

As stated previously, one of the purposes of statistical methods is to summarize large numbers of measurements with a manageable few. To accomplish this task, we must first recognize that the measurements taken on individuals in an investigation are a subset or *sample* of a larger group of individuals who might have been included in the investigation. This larger group is called the *population.* *

If we were able to plot (on a graph) the frequency with which different measurement values occur in the population, we would have a graphical representation of the *population distribution.* A population distribution describes how frequently various data values occur in the larger population from which samples are drawn for observation (Fig. 26-1). Data in this graphical form, however, are difficult to assimilate or communicate.

Rather than describe a population distribution graphically, statistical methods are concerned with a numerical summary of the distribution. Every type of population distribution has a limited number of summary values, called *parameters*, that are used to completely describe the particular distribution of measurements. For example, to completely describe a *Gaussian distribution,* † two parameters are needed: the *mean* ** (the distribution's location along a continuum or, more specifically, its "center of gravity") and the *standard deviation* ‡ (the *dispersion* or spread of the distribution as indicated by how far from the mean individual measurements occur). Figure 26-2 shows a Gaussian

---

* In medicine, we usually think of measurements being taken on persons rather than on animals or objects. This might lead us to the mistaken impression that the statistical use of the term *population* is the same as its use to describe a politically or geographically distinct collection of persons. Although a statistical population might be that type of collection, it is not limited to such. Rather, a *statistical population* is defined as the collection of all possible measurements (not necessarily of persons) from which a sample is selected.

† The Gaussian distribution is also known as the *normal* distribution. We will avoid use of the latter term since *normal* has an alternative meaning in medicine. The Gaussian distribution is the most commonly assumed population distribution in statistics.

** Often you will encounter the term *average* used as a synonym for the mean. In statistical terminology, these are not the same thing. A mean is calculated by summing all the measurements and dividing by the number of measurements. An average, on the other hand, is calculated by multiplying each of the measurements by particular values, called *weights*, before summing them. That sum is then divided by the sum of the weights. A mean is a special type of average in which the weight for every measurement is equal to 1.

‡ The standard deviation (σ) is the square root of the variance (σ^2). The variance is equal to the average square deviation of data (X_i) from the mean (μ). Therefore, the

population standard deviation is equal to $\sigma = \sqrt{\dfrac{\Sigma (X_i - \mu)^2}{N}}$.

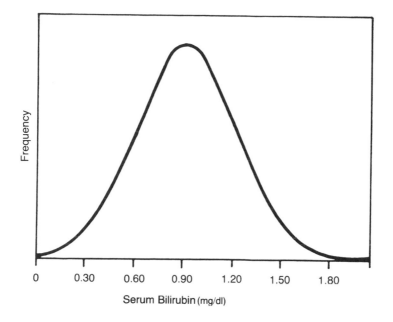

FIGURE 26-1 *A hypothetical population distribution for serum bilirubin measurements.*

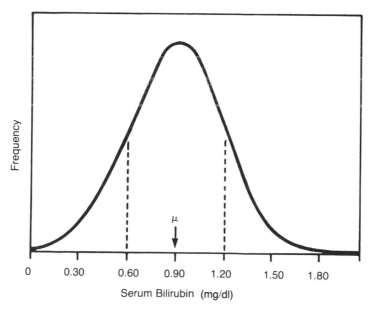

FIGURE 26-2 *A hypothetical Gaussian distribution of serum bilirubin with a mean of 0.9 mg/dl and a standard deviation of 0.3 mg/dl. The broken lines indicate values equal to the mean ± standard deviation.*

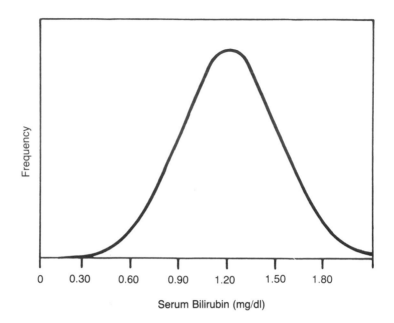

FIGURE 26-3 *A hypothetical Gaussian distribution of serum bilirubin with a mean of 1.2 mg/dl and a standard deviation of 0.3 mg/dl. Comparison of this distribution with that of Figure 26-2 shows what is meant by different locations of population distributions.*

distribution with the mean indicated as the measure of location of the distribution and the standard deviation as the measure of dispersion.

To demonstrate what is meant by the location of a distribution, let us assume that the mean serum bilirubin in the population is 1.2 mg/dl instead of 0.9 mg/dl. The Gaussian distribution of serum bilirubin would then be as shown in Figure 26-3.

Notice that the general shape of the distribution in Figure 26-3 is unchanged by changing the mean, but the position of the center of gravity of the distribution is moved 0.3 mg/dl to the right. If we were to change the dispersion of the distribution in Figure 26-2, however, the shape of the distribution would be altered without changing its position. For example, compare the distribution in Figure 26-2 to Figure 26-4 in which the standard deviation has been changed from 0.3 mg/dl to 0.4 mg/dl.

ESTIMATION AND INFERENCE

We seldom are able to observe all the possible measurements in a population. Using measurements observed in a sample from the

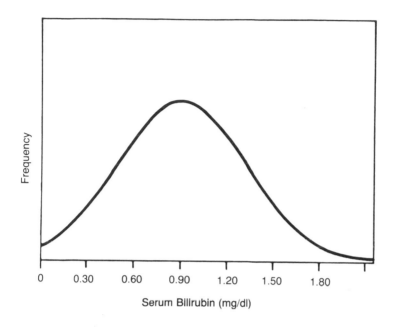

FIGURE 26-4 *A hypothetical Gaussian distribution of serum bilirubin with a mean of 0.9 mg/dl. Comparison of the distribution with that of Figure 26-2 shows what is meant by different dispersions of population distributions.*

larger population, however, we can calculate numerical values to *estimate* the value of the larger population's parameters. These sample estimates of population parameters are the focus of statistical methods. In fact, those estimates are called *statistics!* A single statistic used to estimate the numerical value of a particular population parameter is further known as a *point estimate.* These point estimates are the statistics we use to summarize great numbers of measurements in a manageable few.

Thus far, we have considered only the first purpose of statistical methods: to summarize observations. It is an important step, however, to appreciate the influence of chance on those observations. As stated previously, a sample is a subset of all possible measurements from a population. For *all* statistical methods, it is assumed that the sample is a *random* subset of the population from which it is derived. Although random subsets can be obtained in several ways, in *Selecting a Statistic* we will consider only the simplest (and most common), called a *simple random sample.* In a simple random sample, all measurements in the population have an equal probability of being included in the sample.* Chance, then, dictates which of those measurements are actually included.

When population parameters are estimated using sample statistics, chance selection of the particular measurements actually included in the sample influences how close the sample estimate is to the actual numerical value of the population parameter. Unfortunately, we can never know how close a particular statistic is to correctly reflecting its corresponding population parameter since we would have to measure the entire population to know the actual parameter values. What we can know, however, is how much statistics are expected to vary, based on chance variations among random samples, from a hypothetical value for the population parameter. That knowledge forms the basis of *statistical inference* or *statistical significance testing*.

The framework of statistical inference has been described in Part 1 (see pp. 28–37). There it was pointed out that statistical significance testing is performed under the assumption that the null hypothesis is true. The null hypothesis provides us with the hypothetical value to which our observed estimates can be compared.

As discussed in Part 1, the "bottom line" in statistical significance testing is the P value.† P values are calculated from research observations by first converting those observations to a *standard distribution*. We use standard distributions since the P values at any location in these distributions can be obtained from statistical tables. Much of what we consider to be methodology of statistics is related to conversion of observations to a standard distribution.**

As we discussed in Part 1, an alternative to using statistical significance testing to investigate the influence of chance on sample estimates is to calculate an *interval estimate* or *confidence interval*. ‡ Within a confidence interval we have a specified (often 95%) degree of confidence that the larger population's parameter value is included.***

---

*   In a general sense, a *random sample* implies that any one individual in the population has a known probability of being included in the sample. Here, we are limiting those known probabilities to the condition that they are all equal to each other.

†   Recall that the P value is the probability of obtaining a sample at least as different from that indicated by the null hypothesis as the sample actually obtained if the null hypothesis truly describes the population. It is *not*, as often assumed, the probability that chance has influenced the sample observations. That probability is equal to 1 (i.e., we are certain that chance has influenced our observations).

** Examples of standard distributions include the standard normal, Student-t, Chi-square, and F distributions. Those distributions will be discussed in later chapters.

‡   We sometimes see this interval referred to as "confidence limits." In statistical terminology, confidence limits are the numerical values that bound a confidence interval.

*** In classical statistics, an *interval estimate* means that, if we examine an infinite number of samples of the same size, a specified percentage (e.g., 95%) of the

Commonly, confidence intervals are found by algebraically rearranging calculations used to perform statistical significance tests.

When performing statistical significance tests or calculating confidence intervals, a *one-tailed* or a *two-tailed* procedure can be used. A two-tailed statistical significance test or interval estimate is used whenever the researcher is unsure on which side of the parameter value implied by the null hypothesis the population parameter actually occurs. That is the usual circumstance, but occasionally one encounters *one-tailed* statistical significance tests or interval estimates in the medical literature. A one-tailed test or confidence interval is applicable when the investigator is willing to assume that the direction of the effect being studied is known and analysis is concerned only with examination of the size or strength of the effect.

To illustrate the distinction between one- and two-tailed statistical procedures, let us imagine a clinical trial in which we measure diastolic blood pressure for a group of individuals before and after treatment with a new antihypertensive drug. Prior to examination of the data resulting from the study, we might assume in our study hypothesis that diastolic pressure will decrease when patients are on the drug. In other words, we might assume that it would be *impossible* for the drug to cause an increase in diastolic blood pressure. With that assumption, statistical significance testing or interval estimation can be one-tailed and the statistical power of our analysis increased. If, on the other hand, our study hypothesis is that diastolic pressure will change when patients are taking the drug, statistical significance testing or interval estimation should be two-tailed. That is because we consider it to be *possible*, even though it might be unlikely, that a new antihypertensive drug would cause an increase in diastolic blood pressure.

SELECTING STATISTICAL METHODS

Now, let us turn our attention to the selection of specific statistical methods for analysis of medical research data. Before selecting a statistic, we must make two decisions: (1) which is the dependent variable and which is the independent variable(s), and (2) what type of data constitutes each of those variables. First, let us see what we mean by dependent and independent variables.

---

interval estimates would include the population parameter. A more modern view among statisticians is that this is tantamount to assuming that there is a specified chance (e.g., 95%) that the value of the population parameter is included in the interval. The latter interpretation is usually the one of interest to the medical researcher.

A characteristic for which measurements are made in a study is frequently referred to as a *variable*. For example, if we measured age, we could refer to age as one of the variables in our study. Most statistical methods distinguish between *dependent* and *independent* variables. These are indications of the function (or purpose) of a variable in a particular analysis. Usually a collection of variables that is designed to investigate a single study hypothesis will contain only one dependent variable. That dependent variable can be identified as the variable of primary interest or the end point of a study. We wish to test hypotheses or make estimates, or both, about that dependent variable. On the other hand, that collection of variables might contain no, one, or several independent variables. The independent variable(s) determines the characteristic that needs to be taken into account or other conditions in which hypotheses are to be tested and estimates are to be made.

To illustrate the distinction between independent and dependent variables, consider a cohort study in which the relationship between smoking and coronary heart disease is investigated. Suppose only two variables are measured on each individual: smoking (versus not smoking) and coronary heart disease (versus no coronary heart disease). To analyze those data, we first recognize that we are primarily interested in estimating or testing a hypothesis about the annual risk of coronary heart disease. Thus, coronary heart disease is the dependent variable. Further, we wish to compare the risk of coronary heart disease among smokers to the risk among nonsmokers. Hence, smoking status is the independent variable.

The number of independent variables determines the category of statistical methods that are appropriate to use. For instance, if we are interested in estimation of the annual risk of coronary heart disease in a community without regard to smoking status, or any other characteristic of individuals, we would apply statistical procedures known as *univariable analyses*. Those procedures are applicable to a set of observations that contains one dependent variable and no independent variables. To examine the risk of coronary heart disease relative to smoking status, as in the previous example, however, we would use methods of *bivariable analyses*. Those methods are applied to collections of observations with one dependent variable and one independent variable. Finally, if we were interested in the risk of coronary heart disease for individuals of various ages, sexes, and smoking habits, we would apply *multivariable analyses*.* Those methods are

* A common error in the use of statistical terminology is to refer to procedures designed for one dependent variable and more than one independent variable as *multivariate* analyses. That term, however, properly refers to procedures designed for

used for sets of observations that consist of a dependent variable and more than one independent variable such as age, sex, and smoking habit. Multivariable methods are frequently used to accomplish our third goal of statistical methods: to adjust for the influence of confounding variables.

Medical research investigations often include several sets or collections of variables. For example, suppose we have conducted a controlled clinical trial in which subjects received either drug X or a placebo to facilitate recovery from a particular disease. Since we were concerned about the influence of age and sex on recovery (i.e., we were concerned that age and sex differences might be confounding variables), we included them in our research records. Therefore, our study contains four variables: treatment (drug X or placebo), recovery (yes or no), age, and sex. The collection that includes all four variables would have recovery as the variable of interest and, thus, recovery would be the dependent variable. Treatment, age, and sex would be independent variables, reflecting our interest in examining recovery relative to the specific treatment received and the subject's age and sex. Even before testing hypotheses or making estimates about recovery, however, we would likely be interested in whether randomization achieved dissimilar age distributions in the two treatment groups. The collection of variables that would allow us to compare age distributions contains age as the dependent variable and treatment as the independent variable since age is the variable of interest and treatment group is the condition in which we are assessing age. Thus, the decision as to which is the dependent variable and which is the independent variable(s) depends on the question being asked.

TYPES OF DATA

In addition to characterizing the function of variables in an analysis, we must determine the type of data contained in the measurement of each variable to select a statistical procedure. To categorize types of data, the first distinction we make is between *continuous* and *discrete* data.

Continuous data are defined as providing the possibility of observing any of an infinite number of equally spaced numerical values

---

more than one dependent variable. The use of multivariate procedures is, for the most part, rare in medical research. We have not attempted to include multivariate procedures in our flowchart, and we mention them only in their more common application (multivariate nominal dependent variables).

between any two points in its range of measurement. Examples of continuous data include blood pressure, serum cholesterol, age, and weight. For each of those variables, we can choose any two numerical values and imagine additional intermediate measurements that would be, at least theoretically, possible to observe between those values. We might, for instance, consider the ages of 35 and 36 years. We could imagine ages between 35 and 36 that are distinguished by the number of days since a person's thirty-fifth birthday. Additional values could be imagined by considering the number of hours or minutes since that birthday. Theoretically, there is no limit to how finely we can imagine time being measured. Notice, however, that continuous data need not have an infinite range of possible values, but rather, an infinite number of possible values within their range. That range may, and usually does, have a lower and upper boundary. Age is a good example. The lower boundary is at zero, and it is difficult to imagine individuals having ages much beyond 120 years.

Discrete data, on the other hand, can have only a finite or limited number of values in their range of measurement. Examples of discrete data include number of children, stage of disease, and sex. For each of those variables, we can select two values between which it is not possible to imagine other values. For instance, there is no number of children between two and three children that we could imagine observing in a single family.

It might have occurred to you that, in practice, the distinction between continuous and discrete data is often unclear. For one thing, no variables exist for which we can actually measure an infinite number of values.* We solve this problem by recognizing that, if a great number of measurements can be made over the range of possible measurements and if the intervals between measurements are uniform, then those measurements are virtually continuous. This, however, creates another source of confusion in that it allows data that are, even theoretically discrete, to be redefined as continuous. For example, the number of hairs on one's scalp is certainly discrete data: We cannot imagine observing a value between 99,999 and 100,000 hairs. Even so, the number of possible numerical values within the entire range of the number of hairs is very great. Can we consider such a variable to be composed of virtually continuous data? Yes, for most purposes that would be entirely appropriate.

Data can be defined further by their *scale* of measurement. Continuous data are measured on scales, called *ratio* or *interval scales*, † which

---

* For example, we might imagine, but we could not determine blood pressure to, say, picometers of mercury. So, in reality, all data are discrete!

† The distinction between the ratio scale and the interval scale is that the former scale includes a true zero value; the latter does not. Certain types of discrete data, such as

are defined as having a uniform or constant interval between consecutive measurements. Some discrete measurements are made on an *ordinal scale*. Data on an ordinal scale have a specific ranking or ordering, as do continuous data, but the interval between consecutive measurements is not necessarily constant. A common sort of variable measured on an ordinal scale is an ordering known as the *stage of disease*. We know that, say, stage 2 is more advanced than stage 1, but we cannot assert that the difference between those two stages is the same as the difference between stage 3 and stage 2.

If we are unable to apply any ordering to discrete data, then we say that the data were measured on a *nominal scale*. Examples of characteristics composed of nominal scale discrete data are treatment, sex, race, and eye color. Data that we treat as nominal data include measurements with two categories even though they might be considered to have an innate order, since one is clearly better than the other (e.g., dead, alive).

It is important to note that the term nominal variable can be confusing. In its common use, a nominal variable is a characteristic such as sex or race which has two or more potential categories. From a statistical point of view, however, one nominal variable is limited to only two categories. Thus race or eye color should be referred to as nominal data which requires more than one nominal variable. The number of nominal variables is equal to the number of potential categories minus one.

For purposes of selecting a statistical procedure or interpreting the result of such a procedure, it is important to distinguish between three categories of variables:

1. *Continuous variables* (includes continuous data such as age and discrete data that contain a great number of possible values such as number of hairs)
2. *Ordinal variables* (includes ordinal data with at least three but a limited number of possible values such as stages of cancer)
3. *Nominal variables* (includes nominal data that cannot be ordered such as race, and data that can assume only two possible values such as dead/alive)

The order in which those categories are listed above indicates the relative amount of information contained in each type of variable. That is to say, continuous variables contain more information than ordinal

---

counts, have uniform intervals between measurements and, therefore, also are measured in ratio or interval scales. Other types of discrete data, however, are measured either on an ordinal scale or on a nominal scale.

variables, and ordinal variables contain more information than nominal variables. Thus, continuous variables are considered to be at a higher level than ordinal variables and ordinal variables are considered to be at a higher level than nominal variables.

Measurements with a particular level of information can be *rescaled* to a lower level. For example, age (measured in years) is a continuous variable. We could legitimately rescale age to be an ordinal variable by defining persons as being children (0–18 years), young adults (19–30 years), adults (31–45 years), mature adults (46–65 years), or elderly adults (> 65 years). We could rescale age further to be a nominal variable. For instance, we might simply divide persons into two categories: young and old. We cannot, however, rescale variables to a higher level than the one at which they were actually measured.

When we rescale measurements to a lower level, we lose information. That is to say, we have less detail about a characteristic if it is measured on a nominal scale than we do if the same characteristic were measured on an ordinal or continuous scale. For example, we know less about a person when we label her as a mature adult than we do when we say that she is 54 years of age. If an individual were 54-years-old and we measured age on a continuous scale, we could distinguish that person's age from another individual who is 64-years-old. However, if age were recorded on the indicated ordinal scale, we could not recognize a difference in age between those individuals.

Loss of information when rescaled measurements are used in statistical procedures has the consistent effect, all else being equal, of increasing the Type II error rate. That is to say, rescaling to a lower level reduces statistical power, making it harder to establish statistical significance and, thus, reject a false null hypothesis. What we gain by rescaling to a lower level is the ability to circumvent making certain assumptions, such as uniform intervals, about the data that might be required to perform certain statistical tests. Specific examples of tests that require and those that circumvent such assumptions will be described in greater detail in following chapters.

Thus far, we have reviewed the initial steps that must occur in selecting a statistical procedure. These steps are:

1. Identify one dependent variable and all independent variables, if present, based on the study question being asked.
2. Determine for each variable, whether it is continuous, ordinal, or nominal.

Having completed these steps, we are ready to begin the process of selecting a statistic.

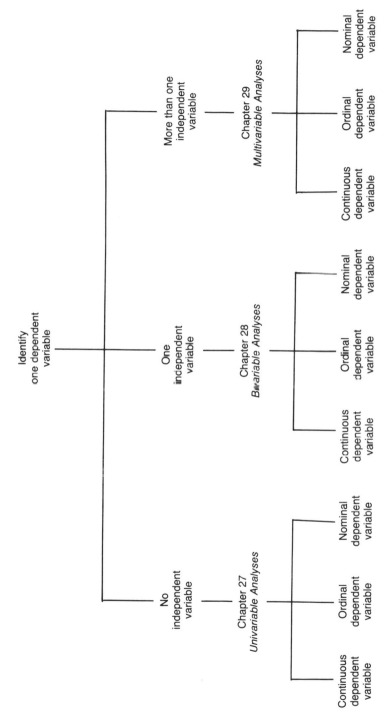

FIGURE 26-5 *Flowchart to determine the chapter and division that discuss statistical procedure relevant to a particular set of variables.*

THE FLOWSHEET

The remaining chapters of this book are arranged as branches of a flowsheet designed to facilitate selection and interpretation of statistical methods. Most, but not all, statistical procedures that might be encountered in medical research have been included.

To use the flowsheet (Fig. 26-5), you must first determine which of a set of variables is the dependent variable. If the set contains more than one dependent variable that you wish to consider simultaneously within the same analysis, perhaps you are interested in multivariate statistics and should consult a statistician. If your collection of variables seems to contain more than one dependent variable, the data most likely address more than one study hypothesis. In that case, the relevant variables for a specific study hypothesis should be considered.

Once a single dependent variable has been identified, you can use the number of independent variables in the investigation to guide you to the chapter that discusses this number of independent variables. Each chapter contains three major divisions. The first is concerned with sets of variables in which the dependent variable is continuous. The second division addresses ordinal dependent variables, and the third addresses nominal dependent variables. Within each of those divisions, techniques for continuous, ordinal, and nominal independent variables, if available, are described. Chapter 30 puts together the flowsheets that were discussed in Chapters 27, 28, and 29.

SUMMARY

In this chapter, we have learned that there are three purposes of statistical methods used to analyze medical research data. The first of those is to summarize data. Distributions of data in large populations are summarized by numerical values called parameters. From random samples we estimate the values of those population parameters with point estimates called statistics.

The second purpose of statistics is to take into account the influence of chance on point estimates calculated from sample observations randomly selected from a larger population. There are two general approaches for considering chance. One of those is statistical significance testing. In this approach, observations on samples are compared to what would be expected if no association between variables or differences between groups exists in the larger population. If the observations are sufficiently unexpected if there is no true association (or differences), we reject the hypothesis that no association (or differences) exists in the larger population. An alternative approach to consider chance is to calculate a confidence interval for the point estimate. In this approach, we can assume, with a specified degree of confidence, that the larger population parameter is included in the confidence interval. Although statistical significance testing and interval estimation are processes with apparently different interpretations, they are simply different mathematical expressions of the same principle.

The third purpose of statistics is to adjust for the effect of confounding variables on our sample observations. This purpose is accomplished in multivariable analysis and will be addressed in Chapter 29.

To accomplish these purposes, we must select a statistical procedure that is appropriate for the study question being asked. To make that selection, we do the following:

1. Decide which variable is the dependent variable. This will be the variable of primary interest in the study hypothesis. The remaining variables are the independent variables.

2. Determine how many independent variables the set of observations contains. If no independent variables exist, we are interested in a univariable procedure. For one independent variable, a bivariable procedure is appropriate. If, on the other hand, the set contains more than one independent variable, we want to use a multivariable method. Remember that for nominal data the number of variables equals the number of potential categories minus one.

3. Define what type of dependent variable is of interest. If the dependent variable can have an unlimited number of equally spaced values, it is a continuous variable. If the dependent variable contains a limited number of values that can be ordered, it is an ordinal variable. A nominal dependent variable simply identifies the presence or absence of a condition.

CHAPTER 27

Univariable Analyses

If a set of measurements contains one dependent variable and no independent variables, the statistical methods used to analyze those measurements are a type of *univariable analysis*. Three common uses of univariable analysis methods are found in the medical literature. The first of these is in descriptive studies (e.g., case series) in which only one sample has been examined. For example, a researcher might present a series of cases of a particular disease, describing various demographic and pathophysiologic measurements on those patients. The purpose of analysis in such a study would be to account for the influence of chance in the measurement of each characteristic. Since there are not separate groups of individuals to be compared and there is no interest in comparing one characteristic with another, each characteristic of persons with the disease is considered a dependent variable in a separate univariable analysis.

The second common application of univariable analysis is when a sample is drawn for inclusion in a study. For example, prior to randomization in a controlled clinical trial, we might wish to perform measurements on the entire sample chosen for study. That is to say, we may wish to determine the mean age and percentage of women in the group selected to be randomized before they are assigned to a study or control group. As in the descriptive study described above, each characteristic that is examined in the sample is a dependent variable in a separate univariable analysis.

Usually, in descriptive studies and when examining one sample, the interest is in point and interval estimation rather than statistical significance testing. Tests of hypotheses are possible in the univariable setting, but one must specify, in the null hypothesis, a value for a population parameter. Often it is not possible to do this in a univariable analysis. For example, it is difficult to imagine what value would be hypothesized for prevalence of hypertension among individuals in a particular community.* However, the third application of univariable analysis is one in which such a hypothesized value is easier to imagine. That is the case in which a measurement, such as diastolic blood pressure, is made twice on the same, or very similar, individuals, and the difference between the measurements is of interest. In that application, it is logical to imagine a null hypothesis stating that the difference between measurements is equal to zero. Thus, the difference in diastolic blood pressure measurements is the dependent variable. Even though the difference, by its nature, is a comparison of groups, differences themselves are *not* compared between any groups. Therefore, there is no independent variable. When comparing two measurements on the same, or very similar, individuals, we are dealing with a univariable problem. Thus, in an investigation using paired data in which each pair constitutes one observation the data are analyzed using univariable methods. The pairs may consist of data from one individual or two individuals who are paired before the data are analyzed.

CONTINUOUS DEPENDENT VARIABLE

In Figure 27-1 we will start by asking, "In which aspect of the population distribution are we interested?" Are we interested in the location of the population distribution or its dispersion?† Next, we must consider the point estimate that might be used to represent that aspect of the population distribution.

In univariable analysis of a continuous dependent variable, data are usually assumed to come from a population with a Gaussian distribution. Therefore, the mean is commonly used to measure location. Dispersion of Gaussian distributions is measured by the standard deviation or, alternatively, by the standard deviation squared, which is called the *variance*. For purposes of analysis, either the variance or the coefficient of variation, as described below, is used to measure the dispersion of the population distribution. Finally, each flowsheet

---

* At first, it might seem that a null hypothesis might be that the prevalence in a particular community is equal to the prevalence in some other community or the prevalence estimated in another study. It is important to keep in mind, however, that the value suggested for a population parameter in a null hypothesis must *be known without error*. That will not be true unless all members of the comparison community were included in the calculation of prevalence.
† In subsequent chapters we will restrict our attention to interest in location.

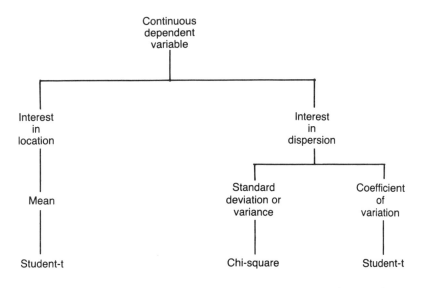

FIGURE 27-1 *Flowchart to select a univariable statistical procedure for a continuous dependent variable (continued from Fig. 26-5).*

will list the general category of statistical techniques that are most frequently used to calculate confidence intervals or test statistical hypotheses.

In Chapter 26 we learned that the first steps in choosing a statistical procedure are:

1. Decide which variable is the dependent variable.
2. Determine how many, if any, independent variables the set of observations contains.
3. Define the type of dependent variable as being continuous, ordinal, or nominal.

To those steps we now add the following:

4. Select the parameter of the population distribution about which we would like to test hypotheses or make estimates. That is, are we interested in location or dispersion?

If we follow those steps on Figure 27-1, we find that we are led to the name of a general class of statistical procedures. Those procedures are usually appropriate for either statistical significance testing or for calculation of confidence intervals.

Interest In Location

As stated previously, the sample mean is an estimate of the location of the population mean. The population mean is often the parameter for which we are interested in making estimates. To calculate a confidence interval for the mean of a sample, the *Student-t distribution* is most often used. The Student-t distribution is a standard distribution to which means of continuous dependent variables are converted to make analysis easier. The Student-t distribution is like the Gaussian distribution, but the Student-t distribution requires an additional parameter known as *degrees of freedom*. The purpose of degrees of freedom in the Student-t distribution is to reflect the role of chance in estimation of the standard deviation.*

The Student-t distribution allows us to derive confidence intervals based on the observed mean and the standard error. In Part 3, it was pointed out that the standard error of a mean gets smaller as the sample size gets bigger. More specifically, the standard error is equal to the standard deviation divided by the square root of the sample size.

The standard error is used with the Student-t distribution in calculation of interval estimates for means of continuous variables. The confidence interval for a mean is equal to the sample's estimate of the mean ± the Student-t value for the desired level of confidence multiplied by the standard error. For a 95%, two-tailed estimate, the Student-t value is approximately equal to 2 for sample sizes of 20 or more. By adding and subtracting a value equal to twice the standard error to the point estimate of the mean, one can determine an *approximate* confidence interval. That is tantamount to saying, with 95% confidence, that the population's mean lies within the interval limited by the sample mean ± two standard errors.† For example, if we read in a research report that the mean ± the standard error for serum cholesterol in a sample is equal to 150 ± 30 mg/dl, we can be 95% confident that the population mean lies within the approximate interval from 120 to 180 mg/dl.

As mentioned previously, there is a special case of a univariable analysis in which statistical significance testing is applicable. The

---

* Use of the Student-t distribution to make interval estimates for means recognizes the fact that the standard deviation is estimated from the sample. That is to say, the standard deviation is not precisely known.
† Other confidence intervals can, likewise, be estimated by considering multiples of the standard error. Approximately two-thirds of possible sample means lie within one standard error of the population mean. More than 99% of possible sample means are included within the range of the population mean ± three standard errors. It is important to remember, however, that we are assuming that the population of all possible means has a Gaussian distribution when applying these interpretations to confidence intervals or their approximations.

most common example of that case is a study in which a continuous dependent variable is measured twice on the same individual. For instance, we might measure blood pressure before and after a patient receives an antihypertensive medication. If our interest is not really in the actual measurements before and after treatment, but rather in the difference between those measurements, we have a *paired design.**
This is a univariable problem since the dependent variable is the difference between measurements and no independent variable exists. By using a paired design, we have attempted to remove the influence of variation between subjects in the initial, or *baseline*, measurement.

A Student-t distribution is used to test hypotheses or construct interval estimates for continuous data from a paired design in the same way that it is used for other univariable analyses. Although the statistical procedures used to analyze data collected in a paired design are no different from other univariable procedures, they are often given separate treatment in introductory statistical texts. In those cases, the procedure for examining the mean difference in data from a paired design is called a *paired* or *matched Student-t test*.

Rather than the sample mean ± the standard error, we often see univariable data presented as the sample mean ± the standard deviation. The sample mean ± the standard error communicates how confident we can be in our estimate of the population mean. The standard error is an indicator of the *dispersion of sample means* that might be obtained by sampling the population. The sample mean ± the standard deviation, however, addresses a different issue. The standard deviation estimates, using the sample data, the *dispersion of measurements* in the larger population. Approximately 95% of the data values in a population distribution occur within the range of the population mean ± two standard deviations.† Therefore, when using univariable statistical procedures for a continuous dependent variable, either we are interested in estimating the location of the population mean and, thus, in the standard error, or we are interested in describing the dispersion of data values and, thus, in the standard deviation.

To illustrate how one chooses between presenting the mean ± the standard deviation and the mean ± the standard error, imagine a study describing a series of cases of a particular disease. Suppose that

---

* Another paired design would be a continuous dependent variable measured on two paired individuals that are similar in that they share characteristics that are thought to influence the magnitude of the dependent variable.

† Also, about two-thirds of the population data occur within the mean ± one standard deviation, and more than 99% occur within the mean ± three standard deviations. To apply those interpretations, we assume that the population's data have a Gaussian distribution.

one of the variables measured on those patients is serum cholesterol. If the purpose of the study is to estimate the serum cholesterol values one might expect to observe among *individual* patients with that disease, the standard deviation should be presented since we are interested in the dispersion or spread of the population data. If, on the other hand, the purpose of the study is to estimate the mean serum cholesterol one might expect to observe in a *collection* of patients with that disease, the standard error (or interval estimate) should be provided since we are interested in the dispersion of sample means randomly obtained from the population.

It is important to recognize the difference in the assumptions we make when interpreting the mean ± the standard error compared to the mean ± the standard deviation. When we use the standard error, we assume a Gaussian distribution of the means of samples randomly obtained from a population. In the case of the mean ± the standard deviation, we assume a Gaussian distribution for the population data itself. This assumption is often true for the mean ± standard error as we shall see if we take large enough samples. The assumption for the mean ± standard deviation, however, often is not true.

If the population data have a Gaussian distribution, so will means of samples from that population have a Gaussian distribution. Even if population data do not have a Gaussian distribution, however, a large series of means obtained by repeated random sampling from the same population will eventually have a Gaussian distribution (Fig. 27-2). The likelihood that means will have a Gaussian distribution increases as the number of observations in each sample increases. This important phenomenon is known as the *central limit theorem* and explains statisticians' interest both in means and in the Gaussian distribution. It also allows medical researchers to use statistical methods that assume a Gaussian distribution to analyze mean values obtained from populations in which the data do not have a Gaussian distribution. This is fortunate since many of the variables of interest in medicine come from populations whose data distributions are not Gaussian.

Interest In Dispersion

By far, the most commonly estimated population parameter in univariable analysis of continuous variables is the mean. However, that is not the only parameter that we might estimate from this type of data, and it is not always the best reflection of our interest in a set of observations. Alternatively, we might be interested in the dispersion of measurements in the population. If so, our interest is in the variance or, equivalently, the square root of the variance: the standard deviation of the population.

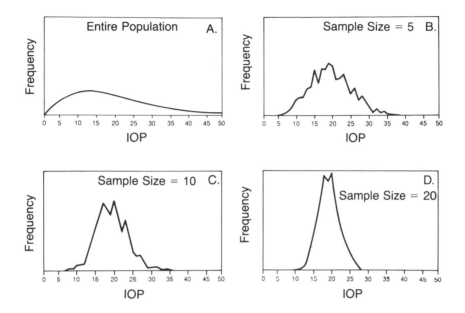

FIGURE 27-2 *Demonstration of the central limit theorem. When we measure intra-ocular pressure for many individuals (A), we find that the distribution of individual measurements does not have a Gaussian distribution. Even so, the distribution of mean intraocular pressure tends to be a Gaussian distribution (B–D). That tendency increases as the size of the sample increases.*

When we are interested in a measure of location of the population from which we have drawn a univariable set of observations, we commonly estimate that location with the sample mean. The standard error addresses the dispersion of sample means. We use the Student-t distribution to test statistical hypotheses or to make interval estimates of the population mean. On the other hand, when we are interested in the dispersion of the population itself, we estimate the population standard deviation or the population variance from our sample observations. If we wish to test statistical hypotheses or calculate confidence intervals for the population variance, we use the *chi-square distribution*. However, use of the variance or standard deviation can be misleading if we wish to compare dispersion among different groups. Let us now take a look at this situation and a common solution.

One of the theoretical properties of the data that have a Gaussian distribution is that the standard deviation and the mean are independent. That is to say, for any particular mean, any standard deviation is equally likely to occur. In practice, this often is not the case. For example, consider body weights from birth through 5 years of age (Table 27-1). It is clear that variation in body weight, as well as body

TABLE 27-1. MEAN AND STANDARD DEVIATION OF BODY WEIGHT
FOR BOYS

| Age (yr) | Weight (kg) | |
	Mean	Standard deviation
Birth	3.50	0.53
1	10.20	1.01
5	18.50	2.17

(From D. S. Smith. *Growth and its Disorders*. Philadelphia: Saunders, 1977).

TABLE 27-2. MEAN AND COEFFICIENT OF VARIATION OF BODY WEIGHT
FOR BOYS

| Age (yr) | Weight (kg) | |
	Mean	Coefficient of variation
Birth	3.50	15.1%
1	10.20	9.9%
5	18.50	11.7%

(From D. S. Smith. *Growth and its Disorders*. Philadelphia: Saunders, 1977).

weight itself, increases with age. That association between the mean
and the standard deviation, however, makes it difficult to compare
measures of dispersion corresponding to different mean weights. For
example, variations of one kg among infants represents much more
variability for their size than does a 1-kg variation among 5-year-olds.

A simple solution to this problem is to divide the standard deviation
by the mean to "adjust" for differences among means. If we multiply
that ratio by 100%, it is known as the *coefficient of variation*. Coefficients
of variation for body weight of boys are presented in Table 27-2.

Examination of the absolute variations in body weight, as estimated
by standard deviations, suggests the least variation among boys at birth
(Table 27-1). That variation, however, is among boys who, on the average, weigh the least. Variation in body weight *relative to the mean* weight
in each group, as estimated by coefficients of variation (Table 27-2),
suggests just the opposite. The variation in weight at birth relative to
total body weight is greater than at any of the other ages considered.

Thus, the coefficient of variation is a useful way to examine the
relative dispersion of continuous dependent variables when it is believed that the mean and the standard deviation are not independent
and we wish to compare univariable estimates of dispersion. Confi-

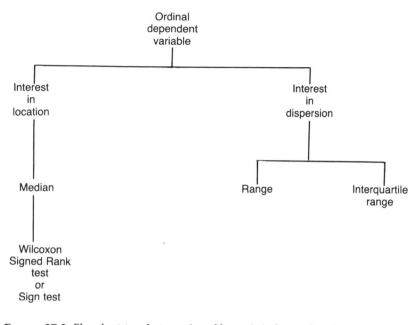

FIGURE 27-3 *Flowchart to select a univarable statistical procedure for an ordinal dependent variable (continued from Fig. 26-5)*

dence intervals and tests of statistical hypotheses for the coefficient of variation use the Student-t distribution.

ORDINAL DEPENDENT VARIABLE

Univariable statistical methods for ordinal dependent variables are presented in Figure 27-3.

Unlike continuous variables, we do not assume a particular distribution of population data, such as a Gaussian distribution, for ordinal variables. Methods used for ordinal variables are, thus, referred to as *distribution-free* or *nonparametric*. It is important to realize, however, that these procedures are not "assumption-free." For example, we continue to assume that our sample is representative of some population of interest.

Interest In Location

Since we are not assuming a particular distribution of population data measured on an ordinal scale, we cannot estimate population parameters that summarize the distribution. We might, however, be interested in describing the location of ordinal data along a continuum. We can do that with the *median*. The median is the mid-point of a collection of data, selected so that half the values are larger and half the values are smaller than the median.

No theoretical population distribution has the median as its measure of location, but it can be used as a *robust** estimate of the mean of a Gaussian distribution. The median circumvents an assumption we make when calculating the mean. That assumption is that intervals between measurements in a distribution are known and uniform. Since the median is calculated using only the relative rank or order of the measurements, the same median would be estimated regardless of whether or not those intervals are known or uniform. Therefore, we can use the median to estimate the mean of a population of continuous data. This is done by ranking sample observations in relative order. The continuous data are, thereby, converted to an ordinal scale by substitution of ranks for the actual measurements.

Strictly speaking, the median can be used as an estimate of the population mean only when the population has a symmetrical distribution. If that is true, the population mean and the population median have the same value (Fig. 27-4). Even though the population distribution is symmetrical, however, it is possible that the observations in a sample obtained from that population are distinctly asymmetrical. A common reason for such asymmetry is the chance inclusion of *outliers* in a sample. Outliers are extreme values that occur in the population with a very low frequency. Occasionally, a sample will include one or more of those extreme values. When this occurs, the sample observations will suggest that these outliers occur with greater frequency than they actually do in the population.

Because the mean is the "center of gravity" of a distribution, its value is influenced more by extreme values than it is by values near the center of the distribution. In those samples that include outliers, therefore, the estimated mean can be quite different from its population value. The sample median, on the other hand, is *resistant* to those outliers. That is to say, extreme values have the same impact on the median as do values that lie closer to the center of a sample distribution. Therefore, paradoxically when a sample from a symmetrical population distribution includes outliers, the sample median is actually a better estimate of the population mean than is the sample mean.

There is, however, a drawback to using the sample median to estimate the population mean. Since the median relies only on the relative ranking of observations, it contains less information than does the

---

* Statistically, a robust estimate is one that is not substantially affected by minor deviations from test assumptions.

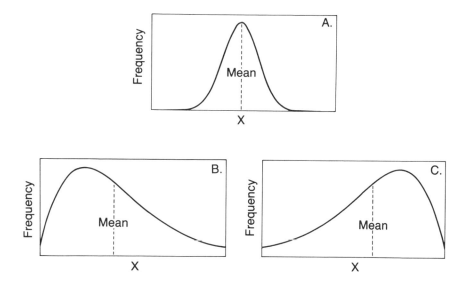

FIGURE 27-4 *Location of the mean for (A) symmetrical and (B, C) asymmetrical distributions. X indicates the location of the median.*

mean. Any time we use less information in statistical procedures, we run a greater risk of making a Type II error. In other words, we have a greater chance of failing to reject an incorrect null hypothesis. We should be willing to run that risk only if we have a reason to suspect that the excluded information would create other, more serious errors if it were included in our data analysis.

Even though the median is used as a robust and resistant estimate of the population mean, it is important to keep in mind that it is also a legitimate measure of the location of a distribution in its own right. For example, if a population distribution is asymmetrical, we might be less interested in the center of gravity or mean of that distribution than we are in its mid-point or median.

If we are interested in testing the null hypothesis that the median is equal to zero in a univariable analysis, we can use either the *Wilcoxon signed rank test* or the *sign test*. Since the median is not a parameter of any particular distribution, we cannot, in general, consider an interval estimate of that parameter. When, however, the median is used as a robust and resistant estimate of the population mean, an interval estimate of that mean is appropriate. Procedures based on the Wilcoxon signed rank test and the sign test are available for such estimation.*

---

* Alternatively, one could calculate a robust and resistant estimate of the standard deviation (described later) and use the Student-t distribution to calculate a confidence interval for the population mean.

Interest In Dispersion

Just as with the sample mean, calculation of the sample standard deviation assumes that intervals between values are known and uniform. The calculation of the standard deviation is greatly influenced by outliers. As an alternative, one often encounters the *range* (difference between the highest value and the lowest value) presented in research reports as a measure of dispersion. Although the range is useful to describe dispersion of a collection of sample observations, it is not a good estimate of the dispersion of population data. This is due to the fact that values at the extremes of most population distributions occur rarely in populations and, thus, rarely in samples. The range is calculated from those extremes, so a range determined from a sample is almost certain to underestimate the population range. Thus, as the size of a sample decreases, the likelihood of observing extreme values decreases. The result is to find sample estimates of the range varying directly with sample size.

As an alternative, the *interquartile range* can be used to describe dispersion of sample observations as well as to estimate dispersion of the larger population. Quartiles divide a distribution into four equal parts, containing an equal number of observations, in the same way that the median divides a distribution into two equal parts. The interval between the data value one quartile below the median and the data value one quartile above the median is known as the interquartile range. Within that interval or range, one-half of the sample data values lie. Since the interquartile range does not depend on extreme values of a distribution, it is much less dependent on the size of the sample than is the range.

For data from a Gaussian distribution, two-thirds of the population values occur within the interval of the mean ± one standard deviation. Therefore, in a Gaussian distribution the population mean ± $2/3$ of the interquartile range can be considered a robust and resistant estimate of the mean ± one standard deviation. If we are concerned about the assumption of known and uniform intervals or if a sample contains extreme values of questionable validity, we can estimate the population standard deviation by calculating two-thirds of the interquartile range instead of using the standard deviation calculated from sample data.

Statistical significance testing and calculation of confidence intervals for the range or the interquartile range are not done. If, on the other hand, the interquartile range is used to estimate the population standard deviation, we may wish to test a statistical hypothesis or to calculate a confidence interval. In that case, we could use the method suggested for measures of dispersion for continuous dependent variables.

NOMINAL DEPENDENT VARIABLE

As the term implies, a *nominal dependent variable* consists only of the name of a particular condition. Further, recall that we limit nominal data to indicators that a condition exists or, by default, that it does not exist. Examples of nominal dependent variables include dead/alive, cured/not cured, and diseased/not diseased. The amount of information contained in a single nominal dependent variable is quite limited compared to continuous dependent variables, such as age, or ordinal dependent variables, such as stage of disease.

When we use nominal dependent variables, we only need to be concerned with measures of location. This might be a surprise since, when we considered continuous and ordinal dependent variables, we discussed the importance of estimates of dispersion as well as estimates of location. For continuous dependent variables, dispersion was an important issue since continuous variables are most often assumed to have a Gaussian population distribution that is characterized, in part, by independence between location and dispersion. That is to say, for a Gaussian distribution, knowing the mean tells us nothing about what the variance of the distribution might be. For any particular mean, any of an infinite number of variances are possible. This is *not* true of the distributions that are relevant to nominal variables. Rather, those distributions have measures of dispersion that are completely dependent on measures of location (which means that they can be calculated from the measure of location or are equal to a constant value). Thus, once we know the measure of location, we know, or can calculate, the measure of dispersion.

The specific univariable statistical method we use to analyze a nominal dependent variable (Fig. 27-5) depends on whether we are dealing with a proportion such as prevalence or a rate such as incidence. Let us first take a look at the methods that are applicable to proportions.

Interest In Proportions

For each measurement or observation of a variable composed of nominal data, we determine only the presence or absence of the condition. For example, we might determine whether an individual in a sample has a particular disease or not. For a sample consisting of more than one observation, we can estimate the *frequency* with which or the number of times the condition occurs in the population. For instance, we can estimate the number of persons in the population with a particular disease. Most often, we are interested in that frequency relative to the number of observations in a sample. If we divide the

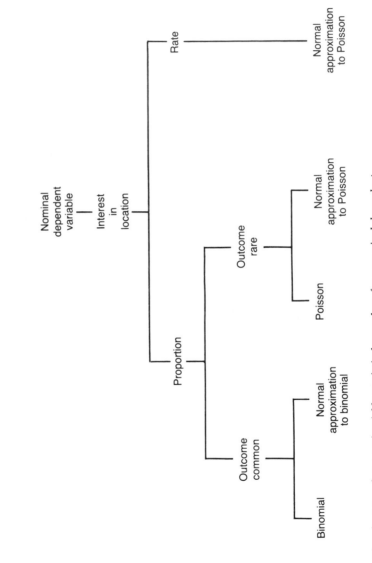

FIGURE 27-5 *Flowchart to select a univariable statistical procedure for a nominal dependent variable (continued from Fig. 26-5).*

number of times a particular condition is observed in a sample by the total number of observations in that sample, we have calculated the *proportion* of observations in the sample with the condition. A proportion calculated from sample observations is a point estimate of the proportion of the population with the condition. An equivalent way to interpret the sample proportion is that it estimates the *probability* of the condition occurring in the population. Two commonly encountered proportions or probabilities in medical research are prevalence and risk. Those measures are discussed in Part 1 and in Part 3.

Probabilities do not have a Gaussian distribution. They are assumed to have either a *binomial* or *Poisson* distribution. A binomial distribution is applicable to any probability calculated from nominal data that meet the following criteria: (1) the probability that any one observation randomly sampled will fall into a particular category, called a *nominal condition* is the same for each observation, and (2) the observations are independent from one another. By *independent*, we mean that the result of one observation does not influence the result of another.

A Poisson distribution is a special case of the binomial distribution in which the nominal event, such as disease or death, is rarely observed, and the number of observations is great. The Poisson distribution is computationally simpler than the binomial distribution. It will, generally, provide a good approximation of the binomial distribution when the number of individuals observed with the condition is less than or equal to 5 and, in addition, the total number of individuals in a sample is greater than or equal to 100.

Statistical significance testing and calculation of confidence intervals for binomial and Poisson distributions are difficult if we wish to perform *exact* procedures that actually use the binomial or Poisson distributions. Fortunately, we do not often have to use exact procedures.

Calculation of confidence intervals or performance of statistical significance tests for nominal dependent variables becomes much simpler when, under certain conditions, the binomial and Poisson distributions can be approximated by the Gaussian distribution. For the binomial and Poisson distributions, we can use a Gaussian approximation, most often called a *normal approximation*, if the number of individuals with a condition is greater than 5 and the number of observations is greater than 10.*

---

* In a normal approximation to a binomial or Poisson distribution, we only need to estimate the probability of observing the event, since the standard error is calculated from that probability. This is unlike using the Gaussian distribution for continuous variables when we must make separate estimates of location and dispersion. As a result, it is not necessary or, in fact, appropriate to use the Student-t distribution to take into account, through degrees of freedom, the precision with which dispersion has been estimated. Rather, the standard normal distribution is used.

Interest In Rates

In statistical terminology, the term *rate* is reserved to refer to a ratio that includes a measure of time in the denominator. This is opposed to the term *proportion*, which includes only the total number of observations in the denominator. The most common measurement of interest in medical research that meets the statistical definition of a rate is incidence.

To illustrate this distinction, imagine that we have observed 100 persons who, at the beginning of our period of observation, were free of a particular disease. At the end of 3 years, 30 of those 100 persons had the disease. If we were interested in the probability that a person randomly selected from the sampled population would develop that disease within a 3-year period, we would calculate the 3-year proportion or risk of disease as 30 per 100 = 0.30. If, however, we were interested in the *rate* at which the disease occurs in the sampled population, we would calculate the incidence of disease as 30/ (100×3) = 0.10 per year. Note that probabilities are unitless, yet rates are expressed in the units of 1/time or events per unit time.

Since diseases usually occur infrequently per unit time, rates are often assumed, in univariable analysis, to have a Poisson distribution. As with proportions, it is possible to perform exact procedures on rates, but more commonly, statistical significance tests and determination of interval estimates for rates rely on a normal approximation. Thus, procedures for rates are the same as those used for probabilities, except that statistical significance testing and interval estimates, if performed, use the Poisson distribution or its normal approximation.

SUMMARY

In this chapter we discussed only univariable procedures. Those methods are used when a set of observations contains one dependent variable and no independent variables. For the most part, univariable analysis is concerned with the calculation of confidence intervals rather than tests of statistical hypotheses. An exception to this is when we have measured a continuous dependent variable twice on the same or very similar individuals. In that case, the dependent variable is the difference between the two measurements. A statistical significance test is usually desired for such paired or matched data to test the null hypothesis that the difference is equal to zero.

During our discussion of univariable analysis of continuous dependent variables, we examined several important principles of analysis of continuous data. One of those, the central limit theorem, gave us some insight as to why statistical procedures for means are so often based on the Gaussian distribution. The central limit theorem says that means tend to have Gaussian distribution even if the population data from which they are derived do not.

Another important principle is the distinction between two measures of dispersion: the standard deviation and the standard error. The standard deviation is a measure of the dispersion of data values in the population. We use the mean plus and minus the standard deviation when we are interested in communicating how much individual observations are expected to vary from one another. The standard error, on the other hand, is a measure of the dispersion of means from samples derived from the population. We use the mean plus and minus the standard error when we are interested in showing how much sample means are expected to differ. It is the standard error that we use to test statistical hypotheses and to calculate confidence intervals for means.

Statistical significance testing and calculation of confidence intervals for univariable analysis of continuous dependent variables assume that the population from which our sample was drawn has a Gaussian distribution. When we doubt that this is the case, we can convert a continuous dependent variable to an ordinal scale. With an ordinal dependent variable or a continuous dependent variable converted to an ordinal scale, we can perform statistical operations parallel to those discussed for continuous dependent variables, but they do not require that we assume that the population has any particular distribution of data values. Those statistical methods are often called nonparametric methods. Alternatively, we can make estimates of parameters of the Gaussian distribution by converting continuous data to an ordinal scale and using the median as a robust estimate of the mean and two thirds of the interquartile range as a robust estimate of the standard deviation. This approach is useful when a sample contains outliers.

Univariable analysis of nominal dependent variables is different in that we do not make independent estimates of location and dispersion. Estimates of location for nominal dependent variables may be proportions or rates. The types of distributions most often assumed for nominal dependent variables are the binomial and the Poisson distributions. The Poisson distribution is used whenever the condition under study is rare. Analysis can involve those distributions directly or, to make calculations simpler, use normal approximations to those distributions.

CHAPTER 28

Bivariable Analyses

In bivariable analysis, we are concerned with one dependent variable and one independent variable. In addition to determining the type of dependent variable being considered, it is necessary, when choosing an appropriate statistical procedure, to identify the type of independent variable. The criteria for classifying independent variables are the same as those previously discussed for dependent variables.

In Chapter 27 we emphasized estimation rather than statistical significance testing. The reason for that emphasis was that appropriate null hypotheses for univariable analyses are, except for observations from paired samples, difficult to imagine. That limitation does not apply to bivariable or multivariable analyses.

In general, the null hypothesis of no association between the dependent and independent variables is relevant to bivariable analyses. However, a school of thought emphasizes calculation of confidence intervals over statistical significance testing for every sort of statistical analysis. The argument is that medical researchers should be concerned with estimating strengths of relationships and should leave hypothesis testing to those who decide health policy. Regardless of your position on estimation versus statistical significance testing, the medical literature contains a mixture of confidence intervals and tests of hypotheses. Therefore, medical researchers and readers of the medical literature must be prepared to properly interpret both approaches.

As described previously, statistical significance testing and estimation are intimately related. Since confidence intervals are, in most circumstances, simply an algebraic rearrangement of the equation used for statistical significance testing, one can use the information in an interval estimate to test null hypotheses and, conversely, the information from a statistical significance test can be used to construct a confidence interval.

When we are dealing with univariable analysis, we can rely on the following relationship between confidence interval and statistical significance testing. A univariable sample's interval estimate that does not extend beyond the numerical value suggested by that null hypothesis, called the *null value*, indicates that a test of the null hypothesis would be statistically significant. If the interval estimate does extend beyond the null value, then a statistical significance test would not be statistically significant.

For instance, assume that the mean change in diastolic blood pressure before and after intervention in a clinical trial with paired observations is 4 ± 1 mm Hg, where 4 mm Hg is the mean difference, and 1 mm Hg is the standard error of the mean difference. From that information, we can calculate an approximate 95% two-tailed confidence interval equal to the following:

$$4 \pm 2 \ (1) = 2 \text{ to } 6 \text{ mm Hg}$$

One way to interpret that confidence interval is to say that we are 95% sure that the mean difference in the population is somewhere between 2 and 6 mm Hg. If, rather than interval estimation, we were interested in testing the null hypothesis that the population mean difference is equal to zero, we could note that the null value, zero, is *outside* the 95% confidence interval. The fact that the 95% confidence interval does not extend beyond zero tells us that a statistical significance test (with a Type I error rate of 100% − 95% = 5%) would result in rejection of the null hypothesis.

Unfortunately, this relationship does not hold for bivariable statistical significance tests. For example, suppose we take samples of 200 persons from two communities and determine the proportion in each sample that have a particular disease. In this example, disease prevalence is the dependent variable, and community is the independent variable. Now, suppose we find 19 persons in the first sample and 33 persons in the second sample have the disease. Our point estimates for the prevalences of disease in the two communities are thus, 19/200 = 0.095 and 33/200 = 0.165. Using a normal approximation to the binomial distribution, we find that the 95%, univariable two-tailed interval estimate of disease prevalence in the first community is 0.0543 to 0.1356. For the second community, the univariable interval estimate is 0.1136 to 0.2164. Those results are illustrated in Table 28-1.

Even though those univariable confidence intervals overlap, it would be incorrect to assume that, in a *bivariable* statistical significance test, we would fail to reject the null hypothesis that the prevalence of

TABLE 28-1. POINT AND INTERVAL ESTIMATES FOR A HYPOTHETICAL
DISEASE FROM SAMPLES FROM TWO COMMUNITIES

Community	Point estimate	95% Confidence interval
1	0.095	0.0543–0.1356
2	0.165	0.1136–0.2164

disease in the two communities is the same. In fact, if we use an appropriate bivariable test on the data presented in Table 28-1 and allow a 5% chance of making a Type I error, we would reject that null hypothesis that the population prevalences are identical ($P = 0.04$).*

Instead of calculating two univariable confidence intervals for observations such as prevalences of disease in two communities, we can calculate a single bivariable confidence interval for the difference or ratio of the two prevalences. For our previous example of two prevalence estimates, the 95%, two-tailed confidence interval for the difference between the prevalences in community 1 and community 2 is 0.0361 to 0.2999. By noting that the bivariable confidence interval does not extend beyond zero, we could correctly conclude that the corresponding statistical significance test would lead to rejection of the null hypothesis that the prevalence of disease in the two communities is the same. In other words, we can reject the null hypothesis that the difference between the prevalences is equal to zero.

Although we have used an example of a nominal dependent variable to demonstrate the distinction between univariable and bivariable confidence intervals and their relationship to bivariable statistical significance tests, the same principle applies to continuous and ordinal dependent variables. Therefore, we need to be careful not to compare the confidence intervals for the dependent variable in each group as a means of obtaining a bivariable statistical hypothesis test regardless of the type of dependent variable we will be considering. Now, let us take a closer look at questions of interest and the methods we use to address these questions in bivariable analysis.

---

* We can however make certain statements about the relationship between univariable interval estimates and bivariable tests of inference. First, if the univariable *confidence intervals do not overlap*, we can assume that the bivariable test of the null hypothesis that parameters are equal in the sampled populations would lead to its *rejection*. Second, if both univariable *confidence intervals overlap the point estimate* from the other sample, we can assume that a bivariable test of the null hypothesis that parameters are equal in the sampled populations would lead to a *failure to reject* that null hypothesis. Unfortunately, situations in which univariable confidence intervals overlap each other but do not overlap point estimates are commonly encountered and do not provide reliable information about the results of bivariable hypothesis tests.

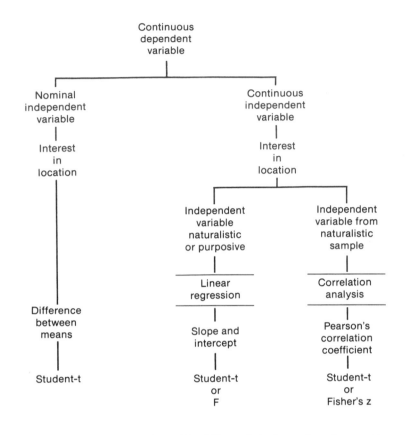

FIGURE 28-1 *Flowchart to select a bivariable statistical procedure for a continuous dependent variable (continued from Fig. 26-5).*

CONTINUOUS DEPENDENT VARIABLE

You might notice two things in examining Figure 28-1. First, you will find that we do not consider a continuous dependent variable associated with an ordinal independent variable. The reason for this omission is that no statistical procedures are available to compare a continuous dependent variable associated with an ordinal independent variable without converting the continuous variable to an ordinal scale. Second, you might realize that we have only included an interest in location. That does not mean that there are no statistical procedures for comparing measures of dispersion; this reflects an almost total interest in location in bivariable and multivariable analysis of medical research data. Methods of comparing measures of dispersion are used to examine assumptions to see if a particular statistical test is appropriate to use with the data. These tests, however, seldom appear in the medical literature.

Nominal Independent Variable

A nominal independent variable divides observations into two groups. For example, suppose we measured bleeding time for women who were birth control pill (BCP) users and nonusers. The dependent variable, bleeding time, is continuous, and the independent variable, BCP use/nonuse, is nominal. A nominal dependent variable divides bleeding time into a group of measurements for BCP users and a group of measurements for BCP nonusers. We have sampled bleeding time from a population that contains a group of BCP users and a group of BCP nonusers.

A universal assumption in statistics is that our observations are the result of random sampling. This assumption applies to the dependent variable, but it is not necessarily assumed by statistical tests for sampling of independent variables.

In general, two methods of sampling independent variables are important to us here.* The first method is called *naturalistic sampling*. In the example of bleeding time, naturalistic sampling would mean that we would randomly select, say, 200 women from a large population and *then* determine who is a BCP user or a BCP nonuser. Then, if our sampling method were unbiased, the relative frequencies of BCP users compared to BCP nonusers in our sample would be repre sentative of the frequency of BCP use in the population.

The second method is called *purposive sampling*. If we used a purposive sample to study bleeding time, we might randomly select 100 women who are BCP users and 100 women who are BCP nonusers. Since the researcher determines the number of observations for each independent variable value, the relative frequency of individuals in the sample with the nominal condition is not representative of the relative sizes of the groups in the population even if our sampling method is random and unbiased. The fact that our sample contains 100 BCP users and BCP nonusers *does not* suggest that half the women in the population use birth control pills.

Thus, the distinction between naturalistic and purposive sampling is whether or not the independent variable in the sample is represen-

---

* There is actually a third method of sampling independent variables. That method is similar to purposive sampling, but instead of selecting observations that have specific independent variable values, the researcher randomly assigns a value, such as a dose, to each subject. This third method of sampling is used in experimental studies.

tative of the distribution of that variable in the population. Naturalistic sampling is most often used in concurrent cohort studies. Purposive sampling is common in case-control and nonconcurrent cohort studies. As we shall see shortly, the method used to sample the independent variable will affect our choice of appropriate statistical techniques or affect the statistical power of the technique chosen.

In bivariable analysis, such as the association between birth control pill use and bleeding time, we are interested in a way in which we can compare bleeding times between BCP users and nonusers. In the comparison of means, our interest is in their difference.* For example, we are interested in the difference between mean bleeding times for BCP users and nonusers. The standard error for the difference between means is calculated from estimates of the variances in the two groups being compared.† To calculate the standard error for the difference in mean bleeding times, we would combine our estimates of the variance in bleeding times among BCP users and the variance among BCP nonusers. Interval estimates and statistical significance testing involving differences between means use the Student-t distribution.

The appropriateness of using the Student-t distribution in statistical significance testing and calculation of confidence intervals is not affected by the method of sampling the independent variable. However, the statistical power of those procedures is greatest when the number of observations is the same for each of the potential categories of the independent variable. That is to say, we would have the greatest chance of demonstrating statistical significance of a true difference in mean bleeding times among 200 women if we used purposive sampling, selecting 100 BCP users and 100 BCP nonusers.

Continuous Independent Variable

We are often interested in using the measurement of a continuous independent variable to estimate the measurement of a dependent variable. As an example, imagine that we are interested in evaluating the relationship between dose of a hypothetical drug for treatment of

---

* The reason for this interest is that differences between means tend to have a Gaussian distribution whereas other arithmetic combinations, such as ratio of means, do not.
† Specifically, this standard error is equal to the square root of the sum of the variances of the distributions of each group mean divided by the sum of the sample sizes. Knowing that, we can more fully understand why we cannot use univariable confidence intervals as a reliable surrogate for bivariable tests of inference. Comparison of univariable confidence intervals is equivalent to adding standard errors of two samples. That is not algebraically equivalent to the standard error of differences between means.

glaucoma and intraocular pressure. Specifically, we would like to estimate the intraocular pressures we expect to be associated, in the population, with various doses of the drug.

Some of the types of questions that can be addressed about estimation of the dependent variable depend on how the continuous independent variable was sampled. Regardless of whether naturalistic or purposive sampling was used, however, we can construct a linear or straight-line equation to estimate the mean value of the dependent variable $(\hat{Y}_i)$ for each value of the independent variable (X_i). In our example, the dependent variable is the mean intraocular pressure, and the independent variable is the dose of medication. A linear equation in a population is described by two parameters: a *slope* (β) and an *intercept* (α).

$$\hat{Y}_i = \alpha + \beta X_1$$

The intercept estimates the mean of the dependent variable when the independent variable is equal to zero. Therefore, the intercept for the linear equation for intraocular pressure and dose would estimate the population mean intraocular pressure for individuals not receiving the drug. The slope of a linear equation tells us the amount the mean of the dependent variable changes for each unit change in the numerical value of the independent variable. For example, the slope of the equation describing intraocular pressure as a function of dose estimates how much intraocular pressure decreases for each unit increase in dose.

If we are interested in this sort of estimation, we need to calculate two point estimates from our sample observations: the sample intercept and the sample slope. To obtain those estimates, we most often use a method called *least squares regression*. This method selects numerical values for the slope and intercept that minimize the distances, or, more specifically, the sum of the differences squared, between the data observed in the sample and those estimated by the linear equation.*

One way to present observations from studies such as the drug and intraocular pressure study is to examine the relationship between intraocular pressure and dose in a *scatterplot* (Fig. 28-2). By convention, the independent variable occupies the *abscissa* or horizontal axis, and the dependent variable is on the *ordinate* or vertical axis. In this

---

* The differences between the observed numerical values of the dependent variables and those estimated by the regression equation are known as *residuals*. Residuals indicate how well the linear equation estimates the dependent variable.

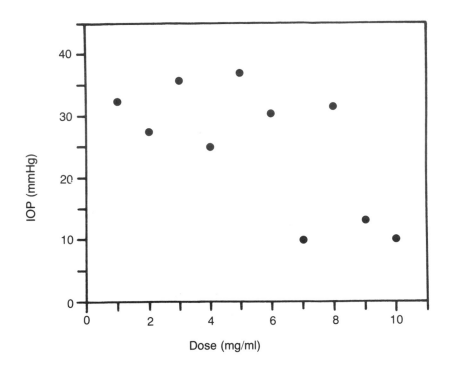

FIGURE 28-2 *Scatterplot of intraocular pressure after treatment with a particular drug at various doses.*

example, we are primarily interested in intraocular pressure; therefore, intraocular pressure is the dependent variable, and dose of the drug is the independent variable.

Using the method of least squares regression, we can estimate the intercept and slope for the relationship between dose (X) and intraocular pressure (Y). We might present estimates of those parameters in a regression equation:

$$\hat{Y}_i = 37.7 + 2.3X_i$$

Additionally, we could present the estimated regression line graphically (Fig. 28-3).

A number of different statistical significance tests and interval estimates are appropriate in regression analysis. For example, we might consider the slope or intercept in separate null hypotheses or calculate

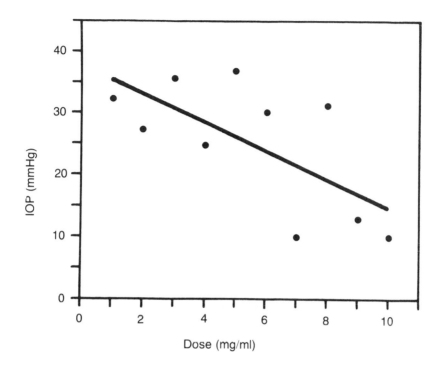

FIGURE 28-3 *Regression of intraocular pressure after treatment with a particular drug as a function of dose.*

confidence intervals for each of those parameters The Student t dis tribution is, most often, used in this application.*

Rather than consider the intercept and the slope separately, how-ever, we can consider the linear equation as a whole. To consider the equation as a whole, we examine the amount of variation in the dependent variable we are *able to explain* using the linear equation divided by the amount of variation that we are *unable to explain* with the linear equation. In the example of medication to treat elevated intraocular pressure, we would divide the variation in ocular pressure

---

* The standard errors of the slope and intercept are functions of the mean of the residuals squared and the dispersion of the independent variable values. The poorer the fit of the linear equation to the observed values of the dependent variable, the lower is the precision with which we can estimate those parameters. On the other hand, the greater the dispersion of the sampled values of the independent variable, the greater is the precision of those estimates. The latter relationship reflects the fact that a straight line can be determined by, at the minimum, two points. The greater the separation of those two points, the more precisely we can define that straight line.

that is explained by knowing medication dose by the variation in intraocular pressure that is left unexplained. Then, we can test the null hypothesis that the regression equation does not allow us to explain the value of the dependent variable, intraocular pressure, given a value of the independent variable, medication dose. We use the F distribution to test that null hypothesis.*

Interval estimation for the linear equation as a whole is usually concerned with confidence intervals around expected means of the dependent variable, such as intraocular pressure, at various values of the independent variable, for instance medication dose. Often, we calculate those interval estimates for all values of the independent variable within the range sampled. Those confidence intervals are presented as a *confidence band* around the regression line (Fig. 28-4).

In extrapolation of study results that have been analyzed with regression methods, we occasionally see speculation about the value of the dependent variable corresponding to values of the independent variable beyond the range of values sampled. For example, we might be tempted to predict intraocular pressure for patients receiving medication doses above or below those included in our study. However, it is dangerous to attempt prediction of mean dependent variable values beyond the sampled range of the independent variable.

One reason for the caution about predicting beyond the range of sampled independent variable values is illustrated by confidence bands. The mean of the dependent variable is most precisely estimated for the mean of the independent variable. This is illustrated for intraocular pressure in Figure 28-4. In that figure, we can see that precision of prediction of intraocular pressure decreases the farther the medication dose value is from the mean dose. That is evidenced by the increasing width of the confidence band in Figure 28-4. If we consider independent variable values beyond the sampled range, the precision with which we can predict the mean of the dependent variable is quite low.

The other reason to avoid this type of extrapolation is that we cannot be sure that the linear equation is applicable for independent variable values for which we have not observed values of the dependent variable. It is possible that low or high doses of the medication fail to conform to the straight-line relationship; they may even work in the opposite direction by raising the intraocular pressure at higher doses.

---

* For regression analysis involving only one independent variable, such as in bivariable regression, the square root of the F statistic used in testing the overall regression is exactly equal to the Student-t statistic obtained when we test the null hypothesis that the slope is equal to zero.

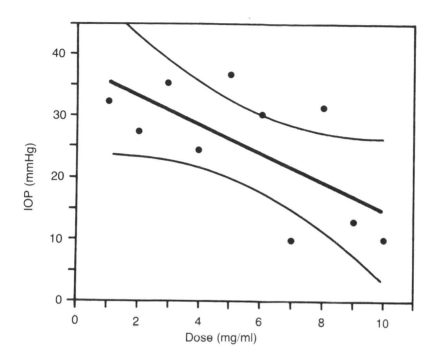

FIGURE 28-4 *Two-tailed 95% confidence band for the prediction of the mean intraocular pressure after treatment with a particular drug from the dose of that drug.*

We make four assumptions when we perform least squares regression. The first assumption, common to all statistical procedures, is that the dependent variable has been sampled randomly. In regression analysis, we assume that random samples of the dependent variable have been taken corresponding to each sampled value of the independent variable. In other words, we assume that we have randomly sampled from the population of intraocular pressures that could result from each of the doses of medication studied.

To determine point estimates of the intercept and slope, we do not have to assume that the random samples come from any particular type of population distribution. When making interval estimates or performing statistical significance testing, however, we assume that the population from which the dependent variable was randomly sampled has a Gaussian distribution at each value of the independent variable. In our example, to calculate the confidence band in Figure

28-4, we assumed that, for each dose studied, intraocular pressure had a Gaussian distribution in the randomly sampled population.

The second assumption in least squares regression is that the spread or dispersion of the dependent variable in the population is the same regardless of the value of the independent variable. That is to say, we assume that the dispersion of intraocular pressure is the same regardless of the medication dose assigned. That equality of dispersion is called *homogeneity of variances* or *homoscedasticity*.

The third assumption is the most obvious and, perhaps, the most critical. To fit a linear equation to observations, we must assume that the relationship between the dependent and independent variables is, in fact, a straight line or linear relationship. For example, we have assumed that a straight line describes the relationship between intraocular pressure and medication dose in the population sampled. Violation of this assumption diminishes the usefulness of linear regression even if all the other assumptions are satisfied.*

The fourth assumption is that the independent variable is measured with perfect precision. In our example, we assume that the medication dose is exactly known. Clearly, this assumption is frequently violated. The effect of its violation is to cause the estimate of the slope from sample observations to be closer to zero than is the true population slope.† Violation of the assumption of a precisely measured independent variable makes it more difficult to reject the null hypothesis that the regression equation does not explain the dependent variable. Therefore, if a regression analysis has failed to demonstrate a statistically significant relationship between the dependent and independent variables, one should ask if measurement of the independent variable might have been sufficiently imprecise to have hidden a true relationship.

---

* Graphical techniques are usually used to test the assumptions of a Gaussian distribution, homoscedasticity, and a linear relationship. If one or more of those assumptions does not appear to be satisfied, one might investigate a *transformation* of the dependent variable. This must be done with caution, however, to ensure that the transformed dependent variable does not violate other assumptions of regression analysis. Alternatively, *weighted regression* procedures sometimes can be employed.
† Why errors in measurement of the independent variable will always cause the slope to be closer to zero is not immediately obvious. To appreciate that this is true, imagine the extreme case in which there is so much error in measurement of the independent variable that it is virtually a random number. For example, in the case of medication dose used to predict intraocular pressure, suppose that the labels on the bottles of medication were misplaced so that we did not know what dose an individual was actually receiving. If we do not know the dosage, we cannot explain intraocular pressure based on dosage. That is to say, we would observe, on the average, no consistent change in intraocular pressure for a unit increase in apparent dose. That situation is represented in a regression equation by a slope of zero. Less extreme errors in assigning dosage would cause us to estimate a population slope somewhere between the actual population value and the extreme value of zero.

In investigations such as the one examining mean intraocular pressure and dose of a medication to treat glaucoma, we usually assign dosages that are not representative of all doses that could have been selected. In other words, we seldom can use naturalistic sampling to investigate a dose-response relationship. It is appropriate to use linear regression methods regardless of whether a naturalistic or a purposive sampling method is used to obtain values of the independent variable. When a representative method of sampling, such as naturalistic sampling, is used to obtain the sample of an independent variable, it is possible to use another category of statistical techniques known as *correlation analysis.*

Correlation analysis might be used, for example, if we randomly sampled individuals from a population and measured both their quantity of salt intake and their diastolic blood pressure. Here, both the independent variable, salt intake, and the dependent variable, diastolic blood pressure, have been randomly sampled from the population. The distribution of quantities of salt intake in our naturalistic sample is representative of the population distribution of salt intake.

The distinction between the dependent and the independent variables is less important in correlation analysis than it is in other sorts of analyses. The same results are obtained in correlation analysis if those functions are reversed. In our example, it does not matter, from a statistical point of view, whether we consider diastolic blood pressure or salt intake as the dependent variable when performing a correlation analysis. However, the same four assumptions as those discussed for the dependent variable in regression analysis are applicable to *both* variables.

In correlation analysis, we measure how the dependent and independent variables change together. In our example, we would measure how consistently an increase in salt intake is associated with an increase in diastolic blood pressure. The statistic that is calculated to reflect how closely the two variables change together is called their *covariance.* The ratio of covariance to the product of the variances of the individual variables is known as the *correlation coefficient* and is symbolized by *r*. The most commonly used correlation coefficient for two continuous variables is known as *Pearson's correlation coefficient.*

The correlation coefficient is a point estimate of the *strength of the association* between two continuous variables. This is an important distinction between regression analysis and correlation analysis. Regression analysis can be used to estimate dependent variable values from independent variable values but does not estimate the strength of the relationship between those variables *in the population.* Correlation analysis estimates the strength of the relationship in the population, but cannot be used to estimate actual values of the dependent variable from values of the independent variable.

The correlation coefficient has a range of possible values from -1 to $+1$. A correlation coefficient of zero indicates no relationship between the dependent and independent variables. *Positive* correlation coefficients indicate that, as the value of the independent variable *increases*, the value of the dependent variable *increases*. *Negative* correlation coefficients indicate that, as the value of the independent variable *increases*, the value of the dependent variable *decreases*.

Interpretation of the strength of association between the dependent and independent variables is facilitated if we square the correlation coefficient to obtain the *coefficient of determination* (R^2). If we multiply the coefficient of determination by 100%, it indicates the percentage of variation in the dependent variable that is explained by or attributed to the value of the independent variable. The coefficient of determination can be thought of as a measure for continuous variables parallel to attributable risk percentage since it addresses how much variability in the dependent variable can be attributed to the independent variable. Remember, however, that it is appropriate to use the coefficient of determination only when the independent variable, as well as the dependent variable, is sampled using representative or naturalistic sampling.

One of the most common errors in interpretation of statistical analysis is to use the coefficient of determination or the correlation coefficient to make point estimates for a particular population even though the independent variable is not sampled by a method that ensures representativeness of its distribution in that population. We can create an artificially high correlation coefficient by sampling only extreme values of the independent variable.

As an illustration of the problem that can occur when interpreting correlation coefficients, let us reconsider the previous example in which we calculated a regression equation to estimate intraocular pressure based on dose of a hypothetical drug for treatment of glaucoma. If we sampled the independent variable, dose, so that we had a uniform representation of doses within the range of 1 to 10 mg/ml as shown previously in Figure 28-2, we would be led to believe that only a moderate negative correlation exists between dose and intraocular pressure ($r = -0.66$). On the other hand, we might decide to limit our study to two levels of the medication and randomly assign five patients to 1 mg/ml and five patients to 10 mg/ml as depicted in Figure 28-5. In that case, we would estimate a much larger negative population correlation coefficient ($r = -0.95$). The estimates for the *regression equation* for both methods of sampling, however, are exactly the same.

To decide which method is representative and, thus, a legitimate use of correlation analysis, we need to anticipate the dosages that will be used in clinical practice. For instance, in clinical practice, will

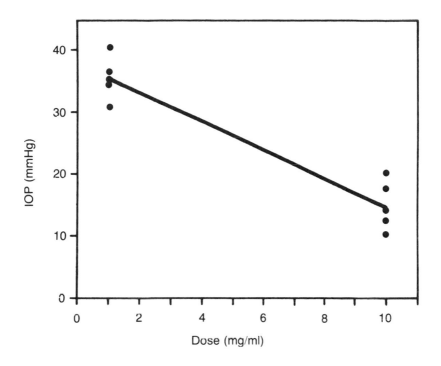

FIGURE 28-5 *Regression of intraocular pressure after treatment with a particular drug as a function of dose when patients are assigned either a dose of 1 mg/ml or a dose of 10 mg/ml.*

patients receive all dosages between 0 and 10 mg/ml with approximately equal frequencies? If so, the correlation coefficient of -0.66 correctly reflects that association between intraocular pressure and dosages that we can expect to experience in practice. If, on the other hand, patients are given dosages of 1 or 10 mg/ml with equal frequency, the correlation coefficient of -0.95 estimates the dose-response relationship that we can anticipate. If any other pattern of drug administration is used in clinical practice, neither correlation coefficient estimates the relationship we might expect between dose and intraocular pressure. For many types of data, it is difficult to choose the applicable independent variable distribution. This is especially true for dose-response relationships. When it is difficult to choose an appropriate independent variable distribution, we can use regression analysis, but correlation analysis should be avoided.

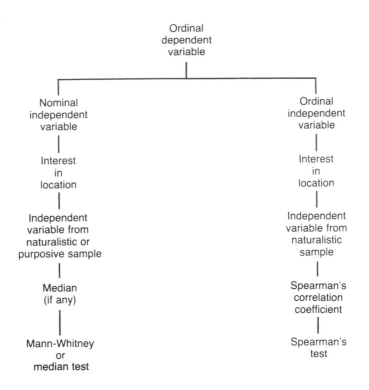

FIGURE 28-6 *Flowchart to select a bivariable statistical procedure for an ordinal dependent variable (continued from Fig. 26-5).*

ORDINAL DEPENDENT VARIABLE

In examination of Figure 28-6, you will find that we do not consider an ordinal dependent variable associated with a continuous independent variable because the continuous independent variable must be converted to the ordinal scale. This is similar to the situation we discussed with a continuous dependent variable included in an analysis with an ordinal independent variable. No statistical procedures are commonly used to compare an ordinal dependent variable with a continuous independent variable without making such a conversion.

Nominal Independent Variable

The *Mann-Whitney test* is a statistical significance test applicable to a nominal independent variable and an ordinal dependent variable. It is also applicable to a continuous dependent variable converted to an ordinal scale to circumvent the assumption of the Student-t test. The null hypothesis considered in a Mann-Whitney test is that the two sampled population groups do not differ in location. Since this is a nonparametric test, no parameter of location is specified in the null hypothesis. Often, we hear the null hypothesis of the Mann-Whitney expressed in a way that concerns equality of medians. This is not far from wrong, but medians of the two sampled groups can be compared more directly in a *median test*.* The median test generally has less statistical power than the Mann-Whitney test.

Ordinal Independent Variable

If the independent variable is ordinal or continuous and converted to an ordinal scale, we can estimate the strength of the association between the dependent and independent variables using a method parallel to correlation analysis. In the case of ordinal variables, the most common correlation coefficient is *Spearman's correlation coefficient*. That coefficient can be calculated without making many of the assumptions necessary to calculate the coefficient described for continuous variables. It is important to remember, however, that *any* correlation coefficient must be determined from samples in which *both* the dependent and the independent variables are representative of a larger population. In other words, we must use naturalistic sampling. There is no nonparametric test that releases us from this assumption.

As for a correlation coefficient calculated for two continuous variables, we can perform statistical significance testing and calculation of confidence intervals for Spearman correlation coefficients. We can also use the square of the Spearman's correlation coefficient to provide a nonparametric estimate of the coefficient of determination or the percentage of the variation in the dependent variable that is explained by the independent variable.

NOMINAL DEPENDENT VARIABLE

Bivariable statistical methods for nominal dependent variables are presented in Figure 28-7.

---

* Even though the median test concerns specific measures of location, it is still a nonparametric test because the medians from the two groups are not assumed to be parameters of any particular population distribution.

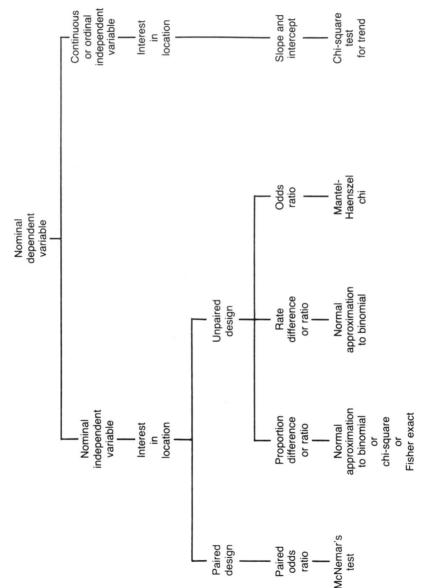

FIGURE 28-7 *Flowchart to select a bivariable statistical procedure for a nominal dependent variable (continued from Fig. 26-5).*

Nominal Independent Variable: Paired Design

If we are interested in collecting information on a nominal dependent variable and a nominal independent variable, we have the choice of a paired or an unpaired design. If appropriately constructed, a paired design may have more statistical power than a corresponding unpaired design. Remember that pairing is the special type of matching in which both the dependent and independent variables are measured on each individual from a pair of two similar individuals and the observations on the pair are analyzed together. When we analyze a nominal dependent variable using a paired design, we use a bivariable procedure rather than using a univariable procedure as we did for a continuous dependent variable from a paired design.

In our previous example of blood pressure measured before and after treatment with an antihypertensive agent, we used a univariable method to examine the difference between blood pressure measurements. With a continuous dependent variable that is measured from paired data, a univariable procedure is appropriate since we can summarize observations from each pair by using the difference in those measurements as the dependent variable. With a nominal dependent variable measured from paired groups, we still are interested in comparing the measurements between pairs, but we cannot summarize nominal data in a way that will allow us to use univariable analysis.

Four possible outcomes among pairs are possible with nominal dependent variables. In two of those outcomes, both members of the pair have the same value for the nominal dependent variable. For example, if survival were the dependent variable in a clinical trial in which individuals were matched or paired as to age and sex before randomizing treatment, both members of the pair might survive or both members of the pair might die. Pairs of that sort are called *concordant pairs*.* The remaining two possible outcomes for nominal independent and dependent variables measured between pairs are those in which the members of the pairs have opposite outcomes. In our example, these outcomes would be when one member of the pair survives and the other member dies. These are known as *discordant pairs*.

Let us consider in more detail the example of a clinical trial to compare mortality between persons who were treated with a particular drug versus those who were treated with a placebo. Suppose we

---

* Concordant pairs are analogous to a difference between pairs equal to zero for a continuous dependent variable in a paired Student-t test. Just as zero does not influence the magnitude of the mean of differences for continuous dependent variables, concordant pairs do not contribute to the evaluation of paired nominal dependent variable interpretation.

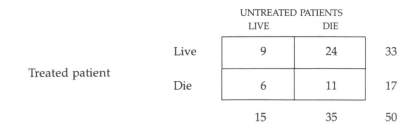

| | | UNTREATED PATIENTS | | |
		LIVE	DIE	
	Live	9	24	33
Treated patient				
	Die	6	11	17
		15	35	50

FIGURE 28-8 *Paired 2 × 2 table for a clinical trial in which mortality is the dependent variable. Patients were randomized by age and sex pairs. Columns indicate the outcome for the untreated member of the pair who received a placebo, and rows indicate the outcome for the treatment member who received a particular drug.*

were concerned about the influence of age and gender on survival, so we identified 50 pairs of patients of the same age and sex and randomized one member of the pair to receive the treatment and one to receive a placebo. Further, imagine that we obtained results from this trial as presented in Figure 28-8. In that case, we would have observed $9 + 11 = 20$ concordant pairs and $6 + 24 = 30$ discordant pairs.

If the treatment in this example had efficacy, we would expect to observe several pairs in which the treated member survived yet the member on the placebo died. Also, we would expect to observe fewer pairs in which the treated member died and the placebo member survived. In other words, we would expect to see a difference between the frequencies of the two types of discordant pairs if there is a difference in the probabilities of surviving between the treated and the untreated patients. Furthermore, the greater the difference between the frequency of discordant pairs, the more efficacy we would estimate the treatment to have.

Rather than examine the *difference* between frequencies of discordant pairs, we usually are interested in the *ratio* of those frequencies. That ratio is an estimate of the population odds ratio. In this example, the odds ratio for paired data is equal to the number of pairs in which the treated member survived and the untreated member died divided by the number of pairs in which the treated member died and the untreated member survived or $24/6 = 4$.

It is important to remember that odds ratios for paired data must be calculated from the discordant pairs. If we were to ignore the fact that the data are paired and act as if the data come from individuals who are not paired, our estimate of the population odds ratio would be inaccurate. To illustrate that point, Figure 28-9 presents the data in Figure 28-8 as if we had analyzed the data assuming we had 100

FIGURE 28-9 *An unpaired 2 × 2 table for the paired data in Figure 28-8. Note how this table differs from the paired table. Here, columns indicate outcomes for individuals, and rows indicate the treatment groups to which the individual was assigned.*

separate individuals rather than 50 pairs. The odds ratio calculated from the data presented in that way is overestimated:

$$\text{Odds ratio} = \frac{33 \times 35}{15 \times 17} = 4.53$$

To conduct statistical significance tests on discordant pairs, *McNemar's test* is used. Related methods can be used to calculate confidence intervals for the odds ratio from paired observations.

Nominal Independent Variable: Unpaired Design

In bivariable analysis of an unpaired nominal dependent variable, as in univariable analysis of nominal dependent variables, we have a choice of whether to measure a proportion such as prevalence, risk, or odds or to measure a rate such as incidence. We also have a choice as to the method of comparing two proportions or two rates. Specifically, we can choose to compare group estimates using either a ratio or a difference of the estimates.

For example, consider a study in which we estimated the prevalence of cataracts among persons exposed to ionizing radiation at a point in time 50 years after their exposure. Suppose, for 50 unexposed persons under 40 years on exposure, the prevalence of cataracts was 2%. For 100 similarly aged persons exposed to a certain level of ionizing radiation, cataract prevalence was approximately 12%. As a point estimate to summarize these data, we might use the prevalence ratio; the prevalence among exposed individuals divided by the prevalence among unexposed individuals, which is equal to 12%/2% = 6. Alternatively, we might calculate the prevalence difference or the

the prevalence among exposed individuals *minus* the prevalence among unexposed individuals, which is equal to 12% − 2% = 10%.

From a statistical point of view, the choice of a ratio or a difference between proportions or rates usually does not matter. In fact, in bivariable analysis, the same methods to calculate confidence intervals and the same statistical significance tests are used regardless of whether the point estimate is a ratio or a difference. This is suggested by the fact that the null hypothesis that a difference is equal to zero is equivalent to the null hypothesis that a ratio is equal to 1. When a ratio is equal to 1, the numerator must be equal to the denominator and, thus the difference between the numerator and the denominator must be equal to zero. In multivariable analysis, however, the distinction between differences and ratios can be very important and will be discussed in Chapter 29.

In bivariable analysis of nominal independent and dependent variables from an unpaired design, we are likely to encounter a variety of statistical methods. As in univariable analysis of a nominal dependent variable, these methods are of two general types: exact methods and normal approximations. The exact method for bivariable proportions is the *Fisher exact* procedure.* Two commonly used approximation methods for proportions are the normal approximation and chi-square procedures.† Rates are most often analyzed using a normal approximation. Statistical significance tests and calculation of confidence intervals for the odds ratio are usually based on the *Mantel-Haenszel chi*, also a normal approximation.**

Continuous Independent Variable

When we have a continuous or ordinal independent variable and a nominal dependent variable, we are able to consider the possibility that a *trend* exists for various values of the independent variable. For example, we might be interested in examining the study hypothesis

---

* The Fisher exact procedure is used when any of the frequencies predicted by the null hypothesis for a 2X2 table are less than five.

† Actually, the normal approximation and the chi-square procedures are equivalent in bivariable analysis. The square root of the chi-square statistic is equal to the normal approximation statistic.

** Frequently, an approximation bivariable statistical significance test for normal variables will involve a "correction for continuity." This is an adjustment to nominal observations when they are converted to a *continuous* distribution, such as the Gaussian distribution, for purposes of analysis. The most familiar example of a continuity correction is Yates' correction used in chi-square analyses. At the present time, statisticians do not agree about the utility of such a correction. Fortunately, the use or disuse of a continuity correction seldom has important impact on the results of analysis.

that the proportion of individuals who develop stroke increases in a linear or straight-line fashion as the diastolic blood pressure increases versus the null hypothesis that no linear relationship exists between those variables. This same sort of hypothesis is considered in simple linear regression with the exception that here we have a nominal dependent variable rather than a continuous dependent variable. Rather than a simple linear regression, we perform a *chi-square test for trend.*

Even though we have a special name for the test used to investigate the possibility of a linear trend in a nominal dependent variable, we should realize that a chi-square test for trend is very similar to a linear regression. In fact, the point estimates in the most commonly used methods to investigate a trend are a slope and intercept of a linear equation that are identical to the estimates we discussed for linear regression.*

Imagine that we are interested in the death rate among persons with stages 1, 2, 3, and 4 cancer. A reasonable study hypothesis might be that the death rate increases as individuals have more advanced stages of cancer. Therefore, we wish to investigate the possibility of a trend in the nominal dependent variable, death rate, with stage of disease. In circumstances such as this in which we have a nominal dependent variable and an ordinal independent variable, it is especially important to remember the fact that a chi-square test for trend is very similar to linear regression analysis. When we look for a trend with an ordinal independent variable, numerical values must be assigned to the ordinal categories.† Just how those numerical values are defined will determine the result of the chi-square test for trend. It is conventional to assign consecutive integers to those ordinal categories unless the categories suggest an alternative numerical scale. Thus, we are actually treating the ordinal variable as if it had equally spaced categories as would occur in continuous data. Fortunately, this is a rather robust test and, therefore, unlikely to be greatly impacted by this assumption violation.**

---

* Point estimation of the coefficients in a chi-square test for trend is identical to estimation in a simple linear regression. For inference and interval estimation, a slightly different assumption is made that causes confidence intervals to be a little wider and P values to be a little larger in the chi-square test compared to linear regression. That difference decreases as the sample size increases.

† Numerical values also must be assigned to the nominal dependent variable, but that choice does not influence the result of inference or interval estimation due to the dichotomous nature of the variable.

** Other methods to examine the trend in a nominal dependent variable for values of an ordinal independent variable that do not require assignment of specific numerical values to ordinal categories have been suggested but do not seem to be as widely used as the one described here. Perhaps one of the reasons for the infrequent use of those alternative methods is that they do not estimate an equation that can be used to examine the relationship between the dependent and independent variables.

SUMMARY

We use bivariable methods to analyze sets of observations that contain one dependent and one independent variable. Independent variables can be continuous, ordinal, or nominal. Nominal independent variables can be thought of as dividing the set of observations into two groups. Estimates of the dependent variable can then be compared between the two groups. In this chapter, we learned that comparison of group estimates in bivariable analysis is not the same as comparing univariable confidence intervals of those variables.

A universal assumption of statistical procedures is that the dependent variable has been sampled randomly. Therefore, we must assume that the distribution of the dependent variable in the sample is representative of its distribution in the population from which the sample was drawn. It is possible for the independent variable to be sampled so that it too is representative of its distribution in the population. Representative sampling of the independent variable is called naturalistic sampling. Alternatively, we can choose the distribution of independent variable values in our sample to maximize statistical power or to ensure the inclusion of levels of the independent variable values that occur rarely in the population. This approach to sampling the independent variable is called purposive sampling. It produces samples with independent variable values that are not representative of the population from which the sample was drawn.

The distinction between naturalistic and purposive sampling is especially important in bivariable analysis of a continuous dependent variable and a continuous independent variable. Here, we are most often interested in estimation of dependent variable values for various values of the independent variable. Actual estimation of dependent variable values is accomplished through regression analysis. The strength of the association between a continuous dependent variable and a continuous independent variable is estimated in correlation analysis. Regression analysis is appropriate regardless of how the independent variable has been sampled. Correlation analysis, however, is useful only when naturalistic sampling has been used to obtain the independent variable.

As in univariable analysis, continuous variables in bivariable data sets can be converted to an ordinal scale if we suspect that the populations from which they have been obtained do not meet the requirements of analyses designed for continuous variables. Methods of analyzing ordinal dependent variables are, for the most part, parallel to analyses for continuous dependent variables. An exception to this is that there is no well accepted method to perform regression analysis on ordinal dependent variables.

Some general principles in bivariable analysis of nominal dependent variables are similar to those for continuous and ordinal dependent variables. In all three, nominal independent variables divide a set of observations into groups to be compared. Further, we are interested in estimation of the dependent variable for various values of the independent variable regardless of the dependent variable type. With nominal dependent variables, this is known as an analysis for trend rather than a regression analysis. The difference in terminology, however, should not be taken to imply that the procedures are very different. In fact, regression analysis performed on a continuous dependent variable is quite similar to the most frequently used method of examining a trend in a nominal dependent variable.

Other general principles in bivariable analysis differ for the three types of dependent variables. One of those is in the analysis of data from a paired design. With a continuous dependent variable, paired data are analyzed using univariable methods. Paired nominal data, however, must be treated with a bivariable method. Another difference is in the way in which point estimates are compared when the independent variable is nominal. For a continuous dependent variable, we compare means between the groups defined by the independent variable by calculating the difference between those means. With nominal dependent variables, however, it is possible to compare proportions or rates either as differences or as ratios in bivariable analyses. The statistical significance tests and calculations of confidence intervals are calculated using the same methods whether differences or ratios are used. Odds, however, are always compared in a ratio.

C H A P T E R 29

Multivariable Analyses

In multivariable statistics we have one dependent variable and two or more independent variables. Those independent variables might be measured on the same scale or on different scales. For example, all the independent variables might be continuous variables or, alternatively, some may be continuous and some nominal variables. We have indicated only nominal and continuous independent variables in the flowcharts that follow. Ordinal independent variables can be considered in multivariable analysis, but they must first be converted to a nominal scale.*

There are three general advantages to using multivariable methods to analyze medical research data. First, this approach allows investigation of the relationship between a dependent variable and an independent variable while "controlling" or "adjusting" for the effect of other independent variables. This is the method of removing the influence of confounding variables in the analysis of medical research data. Thus, multivariable methods are used to accomplish our third and final purpose of statistics in the analysis of medical research results: to adjust for the influence of confounding variables.

For example, if we were interested in diastolic blood pressure for persons receiving various dosages of an antihypertensive drug, we may wish to control for the potential confounding effects of age and sex. To do this in the analysis phase of a research project, we would

---

* Conversion of ordinal scale data to a nominal scale results in a loss of information but needs no justification. Conversion of such data to a continuous scale, however, suggests that the data contain more information than they actually do. This is often difficult to justify.

use multivariable analysis with diastolic blood pressure as the dependent variable and with dose, age, and sex as independent variables.

The second advantage of multivariable statistical methods is that they may allow us to perform statistical significance tests on several variables while maintaining a chosen probability (α) of making a Type I error.* In other words, at times we may use multivariable analysis to avoid the multiple comparison problem introduced in Part 1.

To recall the multiple comparison problem, imagine that we have several independent variables that we compare to a dependent variable using a bivariable method such as the Student-t test. Even though in each of those bivariable tests we permit only a 5% chance of making a Type I error, the chance that we would commit at least one Type I error among all those comparisons would be somewhat greater than 5%. We call the chance of making a Type I error for any particular comparison the *testwise* error rate. The chance of making a Type I error for at least one comparison is known as the *experimentwise* error rate. Bivariable analyses control the testwise error rate. Many multivariable methods, on the other hand, are designed to maintain a consistent experimentwise Type I error rate.

Two types of null hypotheses are examined in most multivariable methods of analysis. The first of those is known as the *omnibus* null hypothesis. That null hypothesis addresses the relationship between the dependent variable and the entire collection of independent variables as a unit. The omnibus null hypothesis is one of the ways in which multivariable methods maintain the experimentwise Type I error rate at $\alpha = 0.05$. A drawback of the omnibus null hypothesis, however, is that it does not allow investigation of relationships between the dependent variable and each of the independent variables individually. That is accomplished by the second type of null hypotheses addressed in *pairwise* or *partial* tests. Those tests do not always maintain an experimentwise Type I error rate equal to $\alpha = 0.05$.

The third advantage of multivariable analysis is that it can be used to compare the separate abilities of two or more independent variables to estimate values of the dependent variable. For example, suppose we conduct a large cohort study to examine risk factors for coronary heart disease. Among the independent variables we measure are diastolic blood pressure and serum cholesterol levels. We would like to determine if both those variables contribute to the risk of coronary heart disease. Examining their ability to explain who will develop coronary heart disease in bivariable analyses, however, could be misleading if individuals with elevated diastolic blood pressure tend to be the same

---

* Since the probability of a Type I error is usually set at 5%, we will use that value in the following discussion.

tend to be the same individuals that have high serum cholesterol. If, on the other hand, we use multivariable methods to compare these risk factors, we would be able to separate their ability to estimate risk of coronary heart disease from their *apparent* association with coronary heart disease due to their association with each other.

Because of these advantages of multivariable methods, they are frequently employed to analyze medical research data. Let us now take a closer look at these methods and the ways in which they can be interpreted to give us these advantages.

CONTINUOUS DEPENDENT VARIABLE

Nominal Independent Variables

In bivariable analysis of a continuous dependent variable and a nominal independent variable, the independent variable has the effect of dividing the dependent variable into two subgroups. In multivariable analysis, we have more than one nominal independent variable and, thus, we are able to define more than two subgroups. The most common methods to compare means of the dependent variable among three or more subgroups are forms of a general statistical approach called *analysis of variance* or, often *ANOVA** (Fig. 29-1).

The simplest type of ANOVA is one in which k nominal independent variables separate the dependent variable into k + 1 subgroups or categories. For example, suppose we are interested in the relationship between fasting blood glucose and race. Further suppose that we define two nominal variables (k = 2) to indicate race: white and black. Those two variables allow us to consider three (k + 1 = 3) subgroups of race for which we determine fasting blood sugar: white, black, and other. This type of ANOVA is known as a *one-way ANOVA.† The omnibus null hypothesis in a one-way ANOVA is that the means of the k + 1 subgroups are all equal to one another. In our example, the omnibus null hypothesis would be that mean fasting blood sugar for whites is the same as for blacks and for persons of other races.

---

* It seems incongruous that a method to compare means should be called an analysis of variance. The reason for that name is that ANOVAs examine the variation between subgroups, assuming that the variation within each of the subgroups is the same. If the variance between subgroups exceeds the variation within those groups, the subgroups must differ in location, measured by means.

† When k = 1, only one nominal independent variable is being considered. In that case, we are comparing only two subgroups, and the one-way ANOVA is exactly the same as a t test for bivariable analysis.

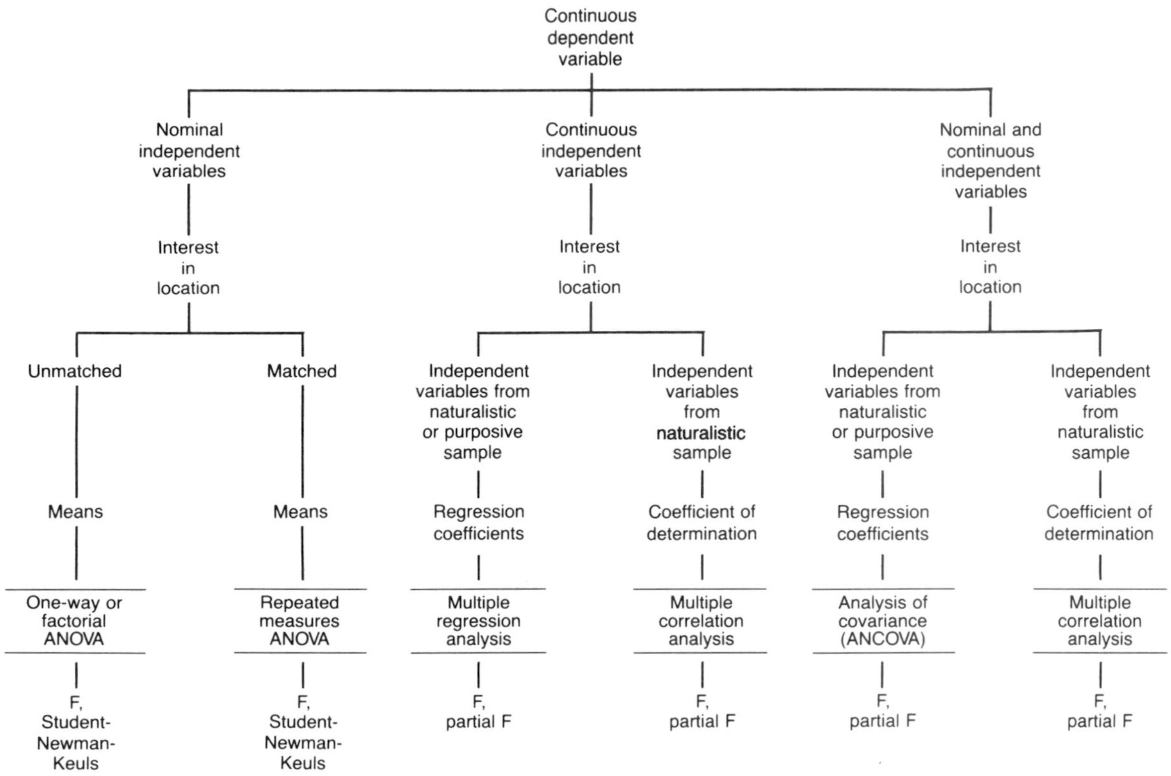

FIGURE 29-1 *Flowchart to select a multivariable statistical procedure for a continuous dependent variable (continued from Fig. 26-5).*

For k nominal independent variables to define k + 1 subgroups, the categories created by the collection of variables must be *mutually exclusive*. By that we mean that it must be impossible for an individual to be included in more than one category. For example, in medical research, we usually regard races to consist of mutually exclusive categories. For each individual, we record a single race category. Thus, it is impossible, in this context, for an individual to be considered both white and black.

When we use a collection of variables such as race and gender, the individual variables are often not mutually exclusive from one another. For example, an individual can be of either gender regardless of his or her race. It is necessary, therefore, to have another way in which subgroups can be defined by nominal independent variables. Commonly, the solution to this problem is found by segregating those variables into *factors*. A factor is a collection of nominal independent variables that defines mutually exclusive, but topically related, categories. For example, suppose we have two independent variables defining race and one independent variable defining gender in our sample of persons for whom we measure fasting blood glucose levels. The three independent variables in this example actually represent two separate factors: race and gender. Instead of k + 1 = 4 subgroups, we define $(k_{race} + 1) \times (k_{gender} + 1) = 6$ subgroups among which we wish to compare mean fasting blood glucose levels: white males, white females, black males, black females, other males, and other females. The type of ANOVA that considers various factors as well as different categories within each factor is known as a *factorial ANOVA*.

In factorial ANOVA, we can test the same sort of omnibus null hypothesis tested in a one way ANOVA. In our example, that null hypothesis would be that mean fasting blood sugar is the same in white females as it is in white males, black females, black males, other females, and other males. In addition, we can test hypotheses about the equality of means of fasting blood sugar between the subgroups within a given factor. That is to say, we can examine the separate effect of race on mean fasting blood sugar or the effect of gender on that dependent variable. The statistical tests that are used to examine the factors separately are often called tests of *main effects*. All these null hypotheses in ANOVAs are tested using the F *distribution*.

The results of examination of a main effect take into account possible confounding relationships of the other independent variable(s). In our example, if we tested the null hypothesis that the fasting blood sugar means for the three race subgroups are all equal by using an ANOVA test of the main effect of race, that test would control for any differences in distribution of genders among those racial groups.

Thus, factorial ANOVA allows us to take advantage of the ability of multivariable analysis to control for confounding variables.

To interpret tests of main effects, it is necessary to assume that the factor has the same relationship with the dependent variable regardless of the level of other factors. That is to say, we assume that the difference between the fasting blood sugar means in blacks, whites, and other races is the same regardless of whether the individual is a male or a female. This is not always the case. For example, females might have a higher fasting blood sugar than do males among white subjects, but females and males might be similar or, in a greater extreme, males might be higher than females in their fasting blood sugars among black subjects. If this sort of relationship exists between factors, we say that an *interaction* exists between gender and race. In medical terminology, we might say that a synergy exists between race and gender in determining fasting blood sugar levels. In addition to testing for main effects, factorial ANOVAs can be used to test hypotheses about interactions.

We have seen how factorial ANOVAs allow us to use the second advantage of multivariable methods by controlling for confounding variables. In our example, we assumed that we were primarily interested in the relationship between race and fasting blood sugar and that we wished to control for the potential confounding effects of gender. An alternative way to think about the data presented in this example might be that we consider race and gender both to be factors that could potentially be used to estimate fasting blood sugar level. In this case, rather than looking at the main effect of race while controlling for gender, we would use the factorial ANOVA to examine how race and gender compare in their relationship to fasting blood sugar. Factorial ANOVAs would, thus, allow us to examine the separate abilities of race and gender to estimate fasting blood sugar. This is an example of the third advantage of multivariable methods.

One-way and factorial ANOVAs are useful methods for sets of observations that include more than one nominal independent variable and a dependent variable that has been measured only once on each individual. This is referred to as an *unmatched* design in Figure 29-1. We know, however, that at times we wish to measure the dependent variable repeatedly on the same individual. We discussed a simple example in Chapter 27 in considering a study in which blood pressure was measured before and after treatment with an antihypertensive medication. In that example, a paired Student-t test was the appropriate method for statistical significance testing and calculation of confidence intervals.

Often, studies in medicine are designed so that they include several repeated measurements of the dependent variable and, perhaps, require control for confounding variables. For example, suppose we are still interested in blood pressure in response to an antihypertensive medication. Now, however, let us imagine that we do not know how long after beginning treatment we can expect blood pressure to stabilize. Thus, we might design a clinical trial in which we measure blood pressure before treatment and once every month for the first year after treatment begins. Since we have more than two measurements of the dependent variable on each individual, we call this a *matched* rather than a paired design. Now, let us further suppose that we are concerned about the potential confounding effects of age and gender. To analyze our observations from that study, we would need a statistical method other than a paired Student-t test. A special ANOVA design allows us to consider several measurements of the dependent variable on each individual and to control for the confounding effects of other variables. That design is known as *repeated measures ANOVA.* *

In ANOVAs designed for both unmatched and matched data, the omnibus null hypothesis maintains an experimentwise Type I error rate equal to α. It is seldom enough, however, to know that differences exist among means within a factor without knowing specifically in which category the means differ. That is to say, it is not enough to know that mean fasting blood sugar differs by race without knowing which races contribute to the difference. To examine the subgroup means in greater detail, we employ pairwise tests.† The most widely used pairwise test for sets of observations that include a continuous dependent variable and more than one nominal independent variable is the *Student-Newman-Keuls test*. That test allows examination of all pairs of subgroup means while maintaining an experimentwise Type I error rate of α = 0.05.** An algebraic rearrangement of the Student-Newman-Keuls test allows calculation of confidence intervals for the dependent variable for each value of the independent variables.

---

* In a repeated measures ANOVA, one of the factors identifies the individual subjects, and the dependent variable is measured for all categories of at least one other factor known as the "repeated" factor. Outside of medical statistics, this design is called *randomized block* ANOVA.

† In ANOVA, these pairwise tests are often called *á posteriori* tests. The reason for that terminology is that some pairwise tests, especially the older tests, require a statistically significant test of the omnibus hypothesis before the pairwise test can be used.

** Other pairwise tests also are available for such comparisons or for different sorts of comparisons among subgroup means. An example of a different type of comparison is one in which we wish to compare a control group with a series of experimental groups.

Continuous Independent Variables

When the independent variables in a study are continuous, we can choose between two approaches that correspond to approaches discussed in Chapter 28 when we considered regression analysis and correlation analysis. Most often, we are interested in estimating values of the dependent variable for all possible independent variable values. In bivariable analysis, we used regression to estimate the value of the dependent variable given the value of the independent variable. When we have more than one continuous independent variable, we can maintain interest in estimation using *multiple regression analysis.*

In multiple regression, the mean of a continuous dependent variable is estimated by a linear equation that is like the one in simple linear regression except that it includes two or more continuous independent variables.

$$\hat{Y} = \alpha + \beta_1 X_1 + \beta_2 X_2 + ... + \beta_k X_k$$

For example, suppose we are interested in estimating plasma cortisol levels based on total white blood cell (WBC) count, body temperature, and urine production in response to a water load. To investigate that relationship, we measure cortisol (μg/100 ml), WBC count (10^3), temperature (°C), and urine production (ml.) in 20 patients. Using multiple regression, we might estimate the following linear equation:

$$\text{Cortisol} = -36.8 + 0.8 \times \text{WBC} + 1.2 \times \text{temperature} + 4.7 \times \text{urine}$$

As in ANOVA, multiple regression allows testing of an omnibus hypothesis that has a Type I error rate equal to α. That hypothesis in multiple regression is that the entire collection of independent variables can *not* be used to estimate values of the dependent variable. An F test is used to evaluate the statistical significance of the multiple regression omnibus null hypothesis. Suppose that, in our example, we find a statistically significant F. This means that, if we know the white blood cell count, temperature, and urine production for a patient, then we can estimate, or make a good guess at, the patient's plasma cortisol level.

In addition to interest in the omnibus hypothesis in multiple regression, it is most often desirable to examine relationships between the dependent variable and individual independent variables.* One way in which those relationships are reflected is in the regression coeffi-

---

* Examination of the relationship between individual independent variables and the dependent variable is analogous to examination of factors in factorial ANOVA.

TABLE 29-1. PARTIAL F TESTS ON REGRESSION COEFFICIENTS ESTIMATED FOR INDEPENDENT VARIABLES USED TO PREDICT PLASMA CORTISOL

Variable	Coefficient	F	P value
WBC	0.8	1.44	0.248
Temperature	1.2	4.51	0.050
Urine	4.7	9.51	0.007

cients associated with the independent variables. Regression coefficients are estimates of the βs in the regression equation. The results of multiple regression analysis allow point estimation and calculation of confidence intervals for those coefficients. Statistical significance testing for individual coefficients involves the *partial F test* to test the null hypothesis that the coefficient is equal to zero. Table 29-1 shows partial F tests for the independent variables used to estimate plasma cortisol. Even though the omnibus hypothesis was rejected in this example, we see that only temperature and urine production have regression coefficients that are statistically significant.

In bivariable regression, the regression coefficients estimate the slope of the line explaining values of the dependent variable as a function of the independent variable in the population which was sampled. In multivariable regression, the relationship between the dependent variable and any particular independent variable is not so straightforward. The regression coefficient actually reflects the relationship between the remaining changes in the numerical values of the independent variable associated with changes in the dependent variable *after changes in the dependent variable associated with changes in values of allthe other independent variables have been taken into account*. That is to say, the reported contribution of any particular independent variable in multiple regression is only the contribution *over and above the contributions of all other independent variables*. This might be considered to be both good news and bad news. The good news is that multiple regression coefficients can be taken to reflect the relationship between the dependent variable and the independent variables "controlling" for the effects of the other independent variables. Thus, multiple regression can be used to remove the effect of a continuous confounding variable.

It might be considered to be bad news that "controlling" for the effect of other independent variables is synonymous with removing variation in the dependent variable that is associated with those other independent variables. If each of two independent variables, by themselves, are good at explaining the same numerical changes in the dependent variable, *both* of those independent variables will appear to be unimportant in explaining changes in the dependent variable in a multiple regression.* If this result is kept in mind, however, multiple regression can be used to examine the separate abilities of the independent variables to explain the dependent variable.

For example, suppose we are interested in cardiac output during exercise. As independent variables, we include energy expended, heart rate, and systolic blood pressure. We know that each of those independent variables is strongly associated with cardiac output. In a multiple regression analysis, however, it would be unlikely that any of them would appear to be statistically significant in their association with the dependent variable. That result is expected to occur because of the large amount of information about cardiac output that is shared by those independent variables.

Calculation of confidence intervals and statistical significance testing for coefficients associated with individual independent variables in multiple regression is parallel to pairwise analyses in ANOVA. In ANOVA, however, pairwise analyses were designed to maintain an experimentwise Type I error rate equal to α. In multiple regression, the testwise Type I error rate is equal to α, but the experimentwise error rate is dependent on the number of independent variables being considered. The more independent variables examined in multiple regression, the greater the likelihood that at least one regression coefficient will appear to be a statistically significant estimator even though no relationship exists between those variables in the larger population being sampled. Therefore, statistically significant associations between the dependent variable and independent variables that were not expected to be important, before the data were examined, should be interpreted with some skepticism.†

If all the continuous independent variables in a set of observations are the result of naturalistic sampling from some population of interest, we might be interested in estimating the strength of the association between the dependent variable and the entire collection of independent variables. This is parallel to our interest in bivariable correlation

---

* Sharing of predictive information by independent variables is known as *multicollinearity*. Some indication of the existence of shared information by independent variables can be obtained by examining bivariable correlation coefficients for those variables, but the best method to evaluate the existence of multicollinearity is to inspect regression models that include and exclude each independent variable. If regression coefficients change substantially when different models are considered, multicollinearity exists.

† This approach to statistical inference and interval estimation is an example of the Bayesian approach. In Bayesian inference, we consider the P value and the prior likelihood, independent of the data, of the null hypothesis being true to determine the likelihood of the null hypothesis in light of the data.

analysis. In multivariable analysis, the method used to measure the degree of association is called multiple correlation analysis. The result of multiple correlation analysis can be expressed either as a multiple coefficient of determination or as its square root, the *multiple correlation coefficient*. It is important to keep in mind that those statistics reflect the degree of association between the dependent variable and the entire collection of independent variables. For instance, suppose that in our example, we obtain a coefficient of determination equal to 0.82, meaning that 82% of the variation in plasma cortisol among patients can be explained by knowing WBC count, temperature, and urine production. The statistically significant F test associated with the test of the omnibus null hypothesis in multiple regression analysis also tests the null hypothesis that the population coefficient of determination is equal to zero. Confidence intervals for coefficients of determination can be derived from these same calculations.

Nominal And Continuous Independent Variables

Often, we are faced with a set of observations in which some of the independent variables are continuous and some are nominal. For example, suppose we were to conduct a study designed to explain cardiac output on the basis of energy output during exercise. Further, we expect the relationship between cardiac output and energy output to be different for the two sexes. In that example, our set of observations would contain cardiac output, a continuous dependent variable; energy output, a continuous independent variable, and gender, a nominal independent variable.

To examine a data set that contains a continuous dependent variable and a mixture of nominal and continuous independent variables, we use an approach called an *analysis of covariance* or ANCOVA. The continuous independent variables in ANCOVA are related to the dependent variable in the same way that continuous independent variables are related to the dependent variable in a multiple regression. The nominal independent variables are related to the dependent variable in the same way nominal independent variables are related to the dependent variable in ANOVA. Therefore, ANCOVA is a hybrid method containing aspects of both multiple regression and ANOVA.

A common use of ANCOVA that is similar to ANOVA is to study how a continuous dependent variable is estimated by a nominal independent variable while controlling for a second variable. In ANCOVA the variable being controlled for is continuous. An example of this is the ability to control for the confounding effects of age when studying the association between a nominal independent variable, such as treatment versus no treatment, and a continuous dependent variable, such as diastolic blood pressure.

Another way to think about ANCOVA is that this method of analysis is a multiple regression method in which some of the independent variables are nominal rather than continuous. To include a nominal independent variable in a multiple regression, we must convert it to a numerical scale. A nominal variable expressed numerically is called an *indicator* or "dummy" variable.*

Frequently, the numerical values associated with a nominal variable are zero and 1. In that case, a value of 1 is arbitrarily assigned to observations in which one of the two potential categories of the nominal variable occurs, and a value of zero is assigned when it does not occur. As an example, if we were to include female gender in a multiple regression, we could assign a value of 1 for female subjects and a value of zero for male subjects.

To see how indicator variables can be interpreted in multiple regression, let us reconsider the previous example in which we have one nominal independent variable to describe gender and one continuous independent variable, energy output, to describe the continuous dependent variable, cardiac output. The multiple regression model for this example may be expressed as follows:

$$\hat{Y} = \alpha + \beta_1 X + \beta_2 I$$

where
$\hat{Y}$ = Cardiac output
X = Energy output
I = Indicator of male gender (1 for females, 0 for males)

Since males are represented by $I = 0$ and zero times β_2 is equal to zero, the multiple regression equation for males is the same as the following bivariable regression equation:

$$\hat{Y} = \alpha + \beta_1 X$$

---

* Even though we can think of ANCOVA as an extension of ANOVA or of multiple regression, that does not mean that the interpretation of ANCOVA is different in those two applications. In the example of cardiac output described as a function of gender and energy output, we could perform an ANCOVA as an ANOVA with a gender factor controlling for the effect of energy output as if it were a confounding variable. Doing so, we would obtain results that were identical to those we would obtain in the regression approach. Actually, ANOVA, ANCOVA, and multiple regression are all examples of the same statistical procedure known as the *general linear model*. An ANOVA can be represented as a multiple regression in which all the independent variables are numerical representations of nominal variables. The "main effects" are measured by the coefficients associated with those indicator variables and the "interactions" are measured by the product of indicator variables. These are also referred to as interactions in regression.

We also can represent the equation for females as a bivariable regression. In this case, the indicator is equal to 1 and $1 \times \beta_2 = \beta_2$. Since β_2 and α are both constants for females, we can describe the relationship between cardiac output and energy output among females as follows:

$$\hat{Y} = (\alpha + \beta_2) + \beta_1 X$$

If we compare the regression equation for males with the equation for females, we can see that the regression coefficient associated with the nominal independent variable (β_2) is equal to the difference between intercepts (cardiac output when energy output is equal to zero) for females and for males.

One problem with using the indicator variable to compare the relationship between cardiac output and energy output among males with that relationship among females is that we must assume that males and females differ only by the intercepts of their individual regression equations. That is to say, we assume that a unit increase in energy output is associated with the same numerical increase in cardiac output among both males and females. This implies that the slope of the relationship between cardiac output and energy output for males is the same as the slope for females. This assumption of equal slopes is often one that we are unwilling to make. When we cannot make this assumption, we can create another type of variable in the multiple regression approach to ANCOVA by multiplying a continuous independent variable by a nominal independent variable that has been converted to a numerical value. This new variable is called an *interaction term*.* In our example, the ANCOVA equation including an interaction term between energy output (X) and gender (I) would be

$$\hat{Y} = \alpha + \beta_1 X + \beta_2 I + \beta_3 X I$$

For male subjects, that equation again is a bivariable regression equation since $I = 0$ so that $0 \times \beta_3 = 0$:

$$\hat{Y} = \alpha + \beta_1 X$$

---

* Interaction terms are not limited to the product of a continuous variable and a nominal variable. Often, we see interactions that are the product of two nominal variables. It also is possible to consider an interaction between two continuous variables, but the interpretation of that product is much more difficult.

For female subjects, since I = 1, the equation is

$$\hat{Y} = (\alpha + \beta_2) + B_1X + B_3X$$

which can be written as

$$\hat{Y} = (\alpha + \beta_2) + (\beta_1 + \beta_3)X$$

The coefficient for the indicator variable (β_2) tells us the difference between intercepts for males and females. The coefficient for the interaction (β_3) tells us the difference between slopes for those two genders. Thus, we have three independent variables: a continuous variable, a nominal variable expressed as an indicator variable, and an interaction variable. In this situation, an ANCOVA is parallel to having a separate bivariable regression for each of the two categories identified by the nominal independent variable. In the example, we were able to estimate separate regression relationships for females and for males. Further, ANCOVA allows us to compare those two bivariable regression equations by testing hypotheses about the regression coefficients for the indicator and interaction variables.

ORDINAL DEPENDENT VARIABLE

In univariable and bivariable analyses, statistical methods are available to analyze ordinal dependent variables and to allow us to convert continuous dependent variables to an ordinal scale when we could not fulfill the assumptions necessary to use the statistical methods designed for continuous dependent variables. This also is true of multivariable methods for ordinal dependent variables.

Ideally, we would like to have methods for ordinal dependent variables that parallel all the important multivariable methods for continuous dependent variables: ANOVA, ANCOVA, and multiple regression. Unfortunately, this is not the case. The only well-accepted multivariable procedures for ordinal dependent variables are ones that can be used as nonparametric equivalents to certain ANOVA designs.* Thus, Figure 29-2 is restricted to methods that can be used *exclusively* with nominal independent variables and an ordinal dependent variable. Ordinal or continuous independent variables must be converted to a nominal scale to use these methods.

---

* Although not in wide use, *ordinal logistic regression* analysis shows promise as a method that might, eventually, gain acceptance as a way to include continuous independent variables in a multivariable analysis of ordinal dependent variables.

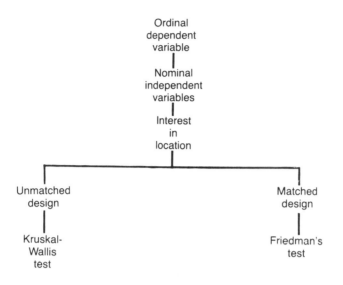

FIGURE 29-2 *Flowchart to select a multivariable statistical procedure for an ordinal dependent variable (continued from Fig. 26-5).*

Let us, for a moment, reconsider the previous example of fasting blood sugar measured among persons of three race categories (black, white, and other) and both genders. In that example, our interest was in determining the independent effects of race and gender on blood sugar. To analyze those data, we used a factorial ANOVA. If we were concerned about fasting blood sugar satisfying the assumptions of the ANOVA,* we could convert those data to an ordinal scale by assigning relative ranks to fasting blood sugar measurements. Then, we could apply the *Kruskal-Wallis test* to those converted data. That test is appropriate for performing statistical significance testing on an ordinal dependent variable and two or more nominal independent variables with either a one-way or factorial design. Nonparametric procedures also are available to make pairwise comparisons among subgroups of the dependent variable.

As previously discussed, statistical methods for ordinal dependent variables are known as nonparametric methods because they do not make assumptions about population parameters. Even so, nonparametric statistical methods test hypotheses relating mainly to the over-

---

* The assumptions for ANOVA and ANCOVA are the same as described previously for regression analysis.

all population distribution. The distinction between parametric and nonparametric hypotheses therefore is that nonparametric hypotheses make statements about the distribution of values for the population in *general* whereas parametric hypotheses make statements about *specific* summary measurements or parameters such as the population mean.

If we are analyzing data from a study in which a continuous dependent variable is measured three or more times on the same individual or matched individuals, we would probably choose a repeated measures ANOVA to analyze our results. If, on the other hand, the dependent variable were ordinal or if it were continuous and we wished to convert it to an ordinal scale to circumvent assumptions of ANOVA, we can still take advantage of the matched design. A nonparametric parallel to a repeated measures ANOVA is *Friedman's test*.

When using multivariable methods designed for ordinal dependent variables to analyze sets of observations that contain a continuous dependent variable that we have converted to an ordinal scale, we should keep in mind a potential disadvantage. This disadvantage is that the nonparametric procedure has less statistical power than does the corresponding parametric procedure if the assumptions of the parametric procedure are not violated by the continuous dependent variable. This is true for all statistical procedures performed on continuous data converted to an ordinal scale. Thus, if the assumptions of a parametric statistical procedure are fulfilled, it is advisable to use that parametric procedure to analyze a continuous dependent variable rather than a parallel nonparametric procedure.

NOMINAL DEPENDENT VARIABLE

In medical research, we are often interested in outcome measurements such as live/die, cure/not cure, or disease/no disease measured as nominal data. Further, because of the complexity of medical phenomena, it is most often desirable to measure several independent variables to consider several separate hypotheses, to control for confounding variables, and to investigate the possibility of synergy or interaction between variables. Consequently, multivariable analyses with nominal dependent variables are frequently used or should be used in the analysis of medical research data.

We have separated multivariable statistical procedures for nominal dependent variables into two groups: those that are useful when the independent variables are all nominal and those that are useful for a

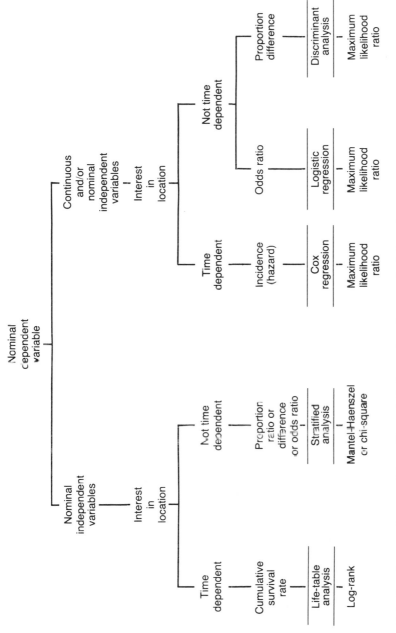

FIGURE 29-3 *Flowchart to select a multivariable statistical procedure for a nominal dependent variable (continued from Fig. 26-5).*

mixture of nominal and continuous independent variables (Fig. 29-3). The analyses in the first group are restricted to nominal independent variables or variables converted to a nominal scale. The analyses in the second group, on the other hand, can be used with nominal and continuous independent variables. There are no well-established methods to consider ordinal independent variables unless they are converted to a nominal scale.

Nominal Independent Variables

When we are analyzing a nominal dependent variable and two or more nominal independent variables, we are interested in measures of location that are the same as those of interest in bivariable analysis of a nominal dependent variable and a nominal independent variable. For example, we might be interested in proportions, rates, or odds. In multivariable analysis of nominal dependent and independent variables, however, we are interested in those measures of disease occurrence while adjusting for the other independent variable(s).

For example, suppose we are interested in comparing the prevalence of lung cancer among coffee drinkers and persons who do not drink coffee. Here, prevalence of lung cancer is the variable of interest and, therefore, the nominal dependent variable. Coffee drinking (yes or no) is the nominal independent variable. Also, we would want to adjust for the potential confounding effect of cigarette smoking. To do that, we might include another nominal independent variable that identified cigarette smokers versus nonsmokers.

When we have two or more independent variables in a data set and they are all nominal, or are converted to a nominal scale, the general approach to adjust for independent variables is often a *stratified analysis*. As described in Part 1, stratified analysis methods involve the separation of observations into subgroups defined by values of the nominal independent variables thought to be confounding variables. In our example of lung cancer prevalence and coffee consumption, we would begin a stratified analysis by dividing our observations into two groups: one composed of smokers and one composed of nonsmokers.

Within each subgroup, such as coffee drinkers and nondrinkers, we would estimate separate prevalences of lung cancer for smokers and nonsmokers. Those separate estimates are known as *stratum-specific* point estimates. The stratum-specific point estimates are combined using a particular system of *weighting* the results from each stratum. That is to say, we would combine the information from each stratum, using one of many methods to determine how much impact each stratum-specific estimate should have on the combined estimate.* The resulting combined estimate is considered to be an adjusted or standardized point estimate for all strata together with the effects of the confounding variable removed.

In the flowchart, we have indicated two types of nominal dependent variables: rates which are *time-dependent* and proportions which are not time-dependent. By time-dependent, we mean that the frequency with which a nominal outcome is observed is dependent on how long persons are followed. For example, consider death as a time-dependent variable. Unless we are studying persons with an unusually high mortality rate, we expect to observe a small proportion of them dying if we were to observe a group for, say, 1 year. On the other hand, if we were to follow those persons for a 20-year period, we would expect to observe a much greater proportion of deaths. Thus far, we have discussed multivariable methods only for nominal dependent variables that are not time-dependent. For example, we have been interested in the prevalence of various conditions. Prevalence is not time-dependent since it refers to the frequency of a condition at a point in time.

Time-dependent variables can cause problems in interpretation if the groups being compared differ in their lengths of follow-up, which is nearly always the case. Those problems can be circumvented if we consider incidence as the dependent variable since the incidence rate has a unit of time in the denominator and, thus, takes length of follow-up into account. Unfortunately, incidence is a measurement that can be confusing to interpret. Most persons find it difficult to intuitively understand what *cases per person-year* means. By contrast, it is much easier to understand *risk*. Recall that risk is the proportion of persons who develop an outcome over a specified period of time. Note, however, that risk is a time-dependent variable since it is determined for a specified period of time. Also, it is not possible to interpret risk calculated from data representing various periods of follow-up as it is for incidence since risk does not contain time in the denominator.

If we are interested in risk and the data contain observations from persons followed for various periods of time, we must use special statistical procedures to adjust for differences in follow-up. When all independent variables are nominal, the methods we use are types of

---

* The system of weighting stratum-specific estimates is an important way in which different stratified analysis methods differ. In direct standardization, the weighting system is based on the relative frequencies of each stratum in some reference population. The most useful weighting systems, from a statistical point of view, are those that reflect the precision of stratum-specific estimates.

life-table analysis. Those methods consider periods of follow-up time, such as 1 year intervals, as a collection of nominal independent variables. Each 1-year interval is used to stratify observations in the same way data are stratified by categories of a confounding variable such as age group. Cumulative survival,* which is equal to 1 minus risk, is determined by combining these adjusted probabilities of surviving each time period.

Two approaches to life-table analysis are commonly used. They are the *Kaplan-Meier* or *product limit* and *Cutler-Ederer* or *actuarial* methods. Those methods differ in how data from persons whose follow-up ended during a time period are handled.† In the Kaplan-Meier method, termination of follow-up is assumed to have occurred at the end of the time block. The Cutler-Ederer method, on the other hand, assumes that the times at which follow-up ended are uniformly distributed during the time period. As a consequence of these different assumptions, Cutler-Ederer estimates of risk tend to be slightly higher than Kaplan-Meier estimates. Statistical methods are available to calculate interval estimates and to perform statistical significance testing for either of those methods.

Continuous And/Or Nominal Independent Variables

The stratified analysis approach that we have been discussing for time-dependent and time-independent nominal dependent variables and nominal independent variables has an appeal to many researchers because it appears to be simpler and more controllable than other sorts of analyses. However, the stratified approach does have some shortcomings. Stratified analysis is designed to examine the relationship between a nominal dependent variable and one nominal independent variable while controlling for the effect of nominal confounding variables. It does not allow for a straightforward examination of alternative explanatory variables, investigation of interactions or synergy, consideration of continuous confounding variables without converting them

---

* Life tables were originally designed to consider the risk of death, but they can be used to calculate the risk of any irreversible outcome.

† Follow-up might be terminated during a time period in life-table analysis in a number of ways. The most common way is due to termination of the study. Often, studies are designed to recruit subjects during most of the study period and to end follow-up at a particular date. Those subjects recruited at the beginning of the study period will contribute data to each of the time periods in a life-table analysis. Those subjects recruited toward the end of the study period will be followed for a shorter period of time and have their follow-up terminated due to completion of the study. Other subjects might be "lost" to follow-up during a time period due to withdrawal from the study, death from a cause not related to the study, and so forth.

to a nominal scale, or estimation of the importance of confounding variables. These are often features of great interest to medical researchers.

Methods of analysis that permit simultaneous investigation of nominal and continuous independent variables and their interactions are parallel in their general approach to multiple regression discussed earlier. The methods we use here, however, are different from multiple regression in three ways. The first difference, as indicated in our flowsheet, is that multiple regression is a method of analyzing continuous dependent variables while we are now concerned with nominal dependent variables. The second difference is that most of the methods for nominal dependent variables do not use the least squares method employed in multiple regression to find the best fit for the data. Most often, nominal dependent variable regression coefficients are estimated using the *maximum likelihood* method.*

The third difference is perhaps the most important to medical researchers interpreting the results of regression analysis of nominal dependent variables. Although this type of analysis provides us with regression coefficient estimates and their standard errors, the remainder of the information resulting from the analysis is unlike that in multiple regression. For one thing, these regressions do not provide us with any estimates parallel to correlation coefficients. Thus, without a coefficient of determination, it is not possible to determine the percent of variation in the dependent variable that is explained by the collection of independent variables.†

For time-dependent outcomes, the most commonly used regression method is the *Cox model.* ** In this approach, the collection of independent variables and, if desired, their interactions, is used to estimate the incidence‡ of the nominal dependent variable*** such as the incidence of death. Simple algebraic combination of the coefficients for a particular Cox model can be used to estimate the survival curve for a set of independent variable values. When all the independent variables are nominal, the Cox model estimates survival curves that are very similar to those resulting from Kaplan-Meier life-table analysis.

---

* The maximum likelihood method chooses estimates for regression coefficients to maximize the likelihood that the data observed would have resulted from sampling a population with those coefficients.
† A surrogate for the coefficient of determination has been proposed, but its usefulness is not well accepted among statisticians.
** This method is also known as *Cox regression* or *proportional hazards regression*.
‡ The term *hazard* is most often used as a synonym for incidence in the Cox model.
*** Actually, Cox regression predicts the natural logarithm of the ratio of the incidence adjusted for the independent variables divided by the incidence unadjusted for those variables.

Thus, increasingly we are seeing the Cox model used in medical research both for the construction of life-table plots and for adjustment for confounding variables.

Nominal dependent variables that are not time-dependent are frequently analyzed using one of two multivariable approaches. These are *discriminant analysis* and *logistic regression.*

As the name implies, discriminant analysis is designed to discriminate between subgroups defined by the nominal dependent variable. Here, we are limiting our interest to analyses that involve one dependent variable, so we are concerned only with discrimination between two subgroups. One of the advantages of discriminant analysis, however, is the ease with which it can be extended to discriminate among more than two subgroups. Thus it can be used with nominal data with more than two potential categories and it then is a mutlivariate statistical method.

Discriminant analysis is very similar to least squares multiple regression,* allowing estimation of a coefficient of determination and related statistics. Regression coefficients estimated in discriminant analysis can be used to predict the probability of membership in a subgroup for individuals with a given set of independent variable values.

Two characteristics of discriminant analysis are, by some statisticians, considered to be shortcomings. Both of those characteristics are related to the fact that discriminant analysis is virtually a multiple regression with a nominal dependent variable. The first of those is that the same assumptions that are required by multiple regression are made for discriminant analysis. Specifically, the concern is with the assumption that the dependent variable has a Gaussian distribution. This is not the case for a nominal variable. Fortunately, multiple regression analysis is a robust procedure allowing its assumptions to be violated to a fair degree before those violations affect the results.

The second concern with discriminant analysis is that it assumes that the probability of subgroup membership is a straight line or linear function. If this is the case, discriminant analysis is the most appropriate method to use. One characteristic of a linear function, however, is that it, theoretically, extends from $-\infty$ to $+\infty$. Since probabilities have a range from 0 to 1, it is possible to predict nonsensical dependent variable values for certain independent variable values. Some statisticians find this potential for impossible predictions to be a disadvantage of discriminant analysis.

As an alternative, nominal dependent variables that are not time-dependent are frequently analyzed using logistic regression. There are three important differences between logistic regression and dis-

---

* In fact, discriminant analysis differs from a least squares regression analysis of a nominal dependent variable only by a constant multiplier.

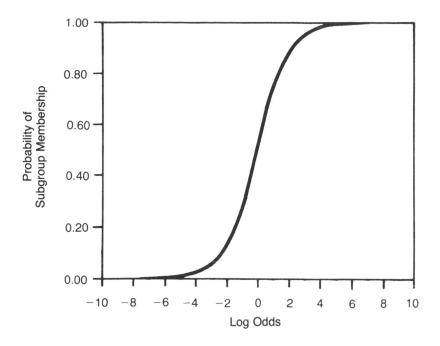

FIGURE 29-4 *An example of a sigmoid curve for the probability of subgroup member-ship determined from log odds.*

criminant analysis. The first is that logistic regression is not so closely related to multiple regression to share the assumption of a Gaussian dependent variable. The second is that the dependent variable is not expressed directly as the probability of group membership. The third difference is that logistic regression techniques cannot readily be extended to consider more than one nominal dependent variable.

The dependent variable in logistic regression is the natural logarithm of the odds of group membership.* With the dependent variable presented in that form, the resulting conversion to estimate probabilities of subgroup membership is confined to the range 0 to 1.† Specifically, those conversions to probabilities follow a *sigmoid* curve within the range of 0 to 1 (Fig. 29-4). Thus, logistic regression satisfies those statisticians who are concerned about discriminant analysis permitting impossible values.**

* This is known as the *logit transformation.*
† Another regression model that has the property of estimating probabilities confined to the range of 0 to 1 is *probit analysis.* Probit analysis is not frequently seen in the medical literature outside of drug trials on laboratory animals.
** There is no assurance, however, that the logistic model is *biologically* appropriate for any particular set of observations. How well the logistic or discriminant models fit a set of observations is determined by the quality of the tests.

TABLE 29-2. REGRESSION COEFFICIENTS FROM A LOGISTIC REGRESSION WITH
OCCURRENCE OF ARCUS SENILIS AS THE DEPENDENT VARIABLE

Variable	Coefficient	P value
Age	0.10	0.002
Sex (female)	1.50	0.030
Cholesterol	0.30	0.010

The regression coefficients that result from logistic regression analysis are often used to estimate odds ratios. Let us see how these odds ratios from logistic regression are interpreted by using an example. Assume that we have conducted a cross-sectional study of a group of persons with arcus senilis and compared them to a group seen by the same ophthalmologist for a refraction. For each subject, suppose we recorded age, sex, and serum cholesterol. Analyzing these data with a logistic regression with the occurrence or nonoccurrence of arcus senilis as the dependent variable, assume we got the logistic regression coefficients shown in Table 29-2.

One thing we can tell from the information in Table 29-2 is that age, sex, and serum cholesterol are all statistically significant estimators of the occurrence of arcus senilis. It is not so easy, however, to interpret the regression coefficients so that we might determine how strongly the odds of having arcus senilis are associated with, say, gender. This becomes easier if we convert those coefficients to odds ratios. For gender, the logistic regression coefficient of 1.50 corresponds to an odds ratio of 4.5. That means that, controlling for the effects of age and cholesterol, women have 4.5 times the odds of having arcus senilis than do men.

We do not normally think of odds ratios for continuous variables. However, the ability to include continuous independent variables is one of the advantages of logistic regression over stratified analyses. The logistic regression coefficients for continuous independent variables can also be interpreted using odds ratios. To do so, we must select an increment in the continuous variable for which an odds ratio can be calculated. For example, we might choose to calculate the odds of arcus senilis for a 10-year increment such as 60-year-olds versus 50-year-olds. In this example, that odds ratio is 2.7. The particular design of logistic regression further means that we would obtain that same odds ratio for *any* 10-year difference in age.

SUMMARY

Multivariable analysis allows us to analyze sets of observations that include more than one independent variable. By providing a method to consider several independent variables at once, the multivariable approach offers three advantages: (1) the effect of confounding variables can be controlled, (2) the multiple comparison problem often can be avoided, and (3) the abilities of independent variables to estimate dependent variable values can be compared.

Multivariable methods for continuous dependent variables are, for the most part, extensions of bivariable analyses that allow more than one independent variable to be considered. For nominal independent variables, the extension of the bivariable Student-t procedure is analysis of variance (ANOVA). In ANOVA we can examine nominal independent variables that indicate various categories of a particular characteristic, or we can look at collections of nominal independent variables known as factors. Two types of null hypotheses can be tested in ANOVA. The omnibus null hypothesis states that all means are equal. The pairwise null hypotheses state that particular pairs of means are equal. Both types of hypotheses are conducted with experimentwise Type I error rate equal to $\alpha = 0.05$ regardless of how many subgroup means are compared.

A special type of ANOVA that is very useful in medical research is known as a repeated measures ANOVA. This procedure is an extension of the univariable Student-t test applied to paired data. Using repeated measures ANOVA we can analyze sets of observations in which the dependent variable has been measured more than twice on the same individual or we may use this method to control for the effect of potential confounding variables, or both.

Associations between a continuous dependent variable and two or more continuous independent variables are investigated with multiple regression analysis, an extension of bivariable linear regression. The ability to consider more than one independent variable in multiple regression analysis permits control of the effect of confounding variables and comparison of the abilities of various independent variables to estimate dependent variable values. Relationships between the independent variables and the dependent variable must be interpreted recognizing that the multiple regression coefficients are influenced by the ability of other independent variables to explain the relationship. Strength of the association between a continuous dependent variable and a collection of continuous independent variables is estimated by the multiple correlation coefficient.

Often, we have a continuous dependent variable, one or more nominal independent variables, and one or more continuous independent variables. Such a set of observations is analyzed with an analysis of covariance (ANCOVA). An ANCOVA has features of both an ANOVA and a multiple regression analysis.

As in bivariable analysis, multivariable methods for ordinal dependent variables can be thought of as nonparametric parallels to procedures for continuous dependent variables. In multivariable analysis, however, parallels for ANOVA methods are the only ones commonly used.

With nominal dependent variables, procedures are either special types of regression analysis or methods that involve stratification. Stratification requires that all the independent variables be nominal or converted to a nominal scale. The regression procedures can involve continuous and nominal dependent variables.

For both types of methods, a further distinction in multivariable analysis of nominal dependent variables is whether or not the measures of location are time-dependent. A stratified technique for dependent variables that are time-dependent is known as life-table analysis. A parallel regression technique is Cox regression. For dependent variables that are not time-dependent, the most common regression method is logistic regression. The coefficients from logistic regression can be reported as odds ratios. Another approach is to use discriminant analysis. One advantage of discriminant analysis is that it can be extended to more than one nominal dependent variable.

CHAPTER 30

Flowchart Summary

In this chapter, we present the entire flowchart that is required for selecting a statistic. This summary flowchart can be used in two ways. One way is to start on page 317 and trace the flowchart forward to discover what types of statistical procedures are appropriate for a particular investigation. To use the flowchart this way, you must first identify one dependent variable and then 0, 1, or more than 1 independent variables. Next, you must decide the type of the dependent variable (i.e , continuous, ordinal, or nominal). After you have made these decisions you will encounter a number that will guide you to the next flowchart element that is applicable to your data.

Each of the subsequent flowchart elements is constructed in a similar way. If your data contains independent variables, you will need to identify their type(s).* Next, for some flowcharts, you have to decide what parameter of the population is of interest to you, location or dispersion.† If special restrictions are applicable to statistical procedures that might be appropriate to your data, you will need to determine if those assumptions or restrictions are satisfied. If the assumptions are not satisfied, you can convert your variable or variables to a lower level scale and consult the flowchart for a flowchart element consistent with your converted variable(s).

---

* Remember that, for statistical purposes, a nominal variable refers to only two categories of a characteristic. If a characteristic has k categories, k-1 nominal variables will be needed.
† The term interest in location is used for bivariable and multivariable analysis as well as univariable where the term has more intuitive meaning. In bivariable and multivariable analysis, we are interested in a measurement which locates the strength of a relationship or size of a difference along a continuum of possible values.

Following down the flowchart, you will come to a summary measurement or point estimate which is useful for your data. These are often followed by a general classification of statistical procedures. At the very bottom, you will encounter the name of the procedures that are most commonly used for both statistical significance testing and calculation of confidence intervals on data sets like yours.

When using the flowchart note that:

1. Measures with a single line under them are point estimates from samples.
2. Procedures with a double line under them are used for statistical significance testing or calculation of confidence intervals.
3. Horizontal lines above and below indicate a class of procedures.
4. When "or" is used it indicates that either test is acceptable for addressing the same question; however the test listed first has more statistical power or is used more frequently, or both.
5. Additional conditions that need to be satisfied to use a type of statistical procedure are shown without lines above or below.
6. When a comma appears between two statistical significance tests, the first test is used to evaluate the omnibus null hypothesis while the second test is used in pairwise comparisons.

That first way of using the flowchart is applicable to persons who are interested in selecting a statistical procedure for a set of data. More often, as readers of the medical literature we are interested in checking that a procedure selected by others is an appropriate one. The flowchart can be used to assist in that process by finding the name of the selected procedure and tracing the flowchart backward to determine if the procedure is a logical choice for the data set being analyzed.

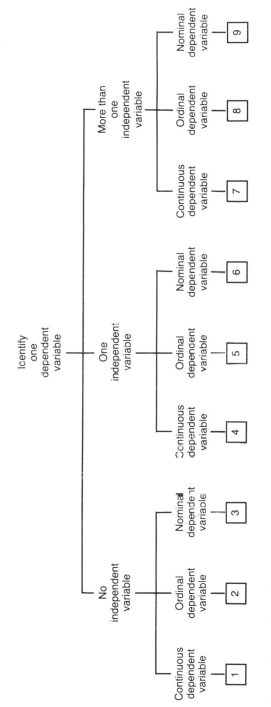

FIGURE 30-1 *Master flowchart to determine which of the subsequent flowcharts are applicable to a particular data set. The numbers at the bottom of the flowchart refer to subsequent flowcharts.*

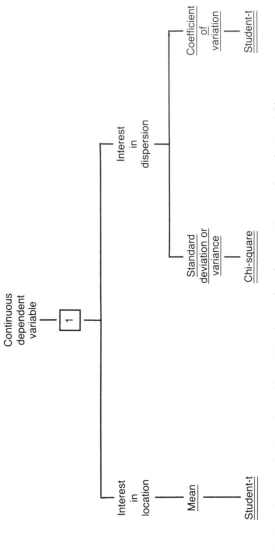

FIGURE 30-2 *Flowchart to select a univariable statistical procedure for a continuous dependent variable.*

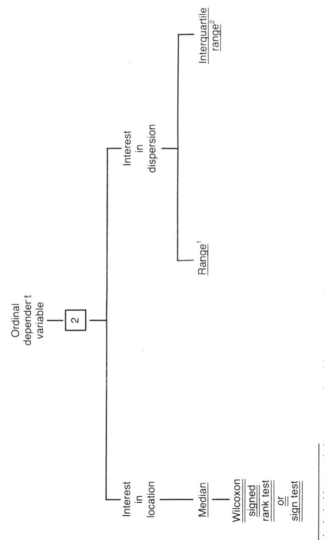

FIGURE 30-3 *Flowchart to select a univariable statistical procedure for an ordinal dependent variable.*

[1]The range is included here only because of its widespread use. It is, however, difficult to interpret as discussed in Chapter 27.
[2]Statistical significance testing and calculation of confidence intervals are not obtained for the interquartile range unless it is used to approximate the standard deviation.

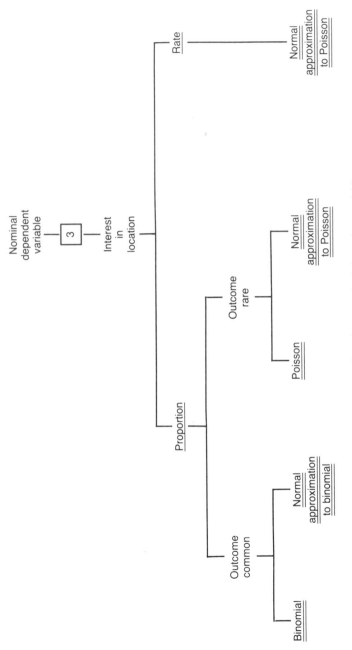

FIGURE 30-4 *Flowchart to select a univariable statistical procedure for a nominal dependent variable.*

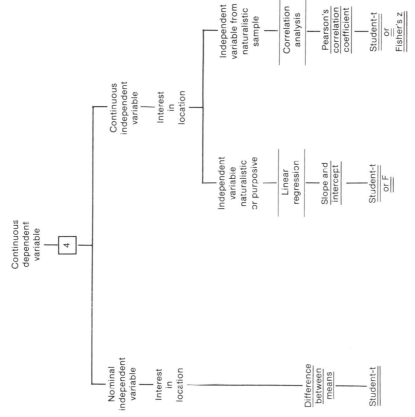

FIGURE 30-5 *Flowchart to select a bivariable statistical procedure for a continuous dependent variable.*

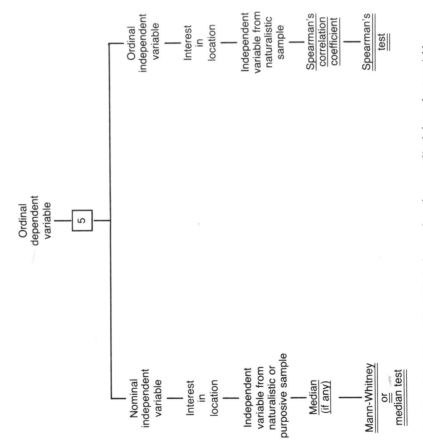

FIGURE 30-6 *Flowchart to select a bivariable statistical procedure for an ordinal dependent variable.*

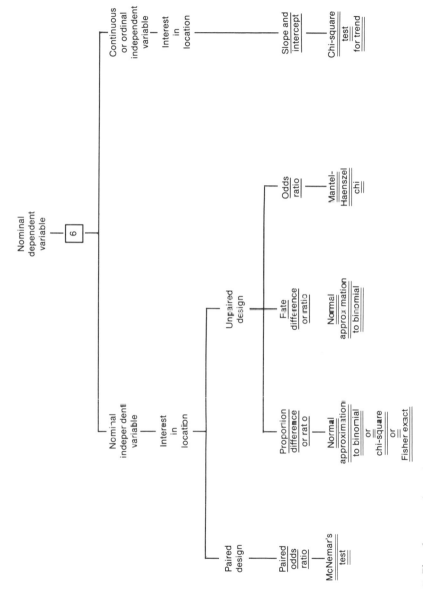

FIGURE 30-7 *Flowchart to select a bivariable statistical procedure for a nominal dependent variable.*

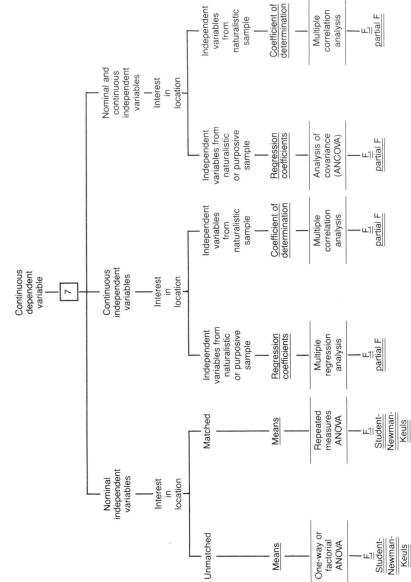

FIGURE 30-8 *Flowchart to select a multivariable statistical procedure for a continuous dependent variable.*

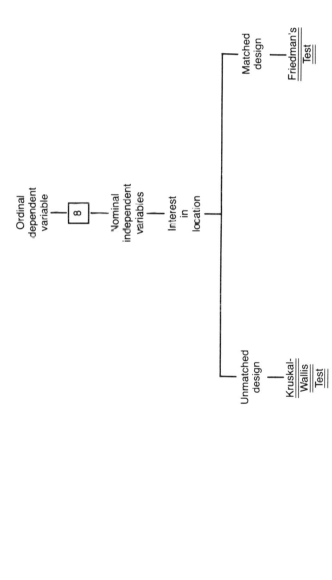

FIGURE 30-9 *Flowchart to select a multivariable statistical procedure for an ordinal dependent variable.*

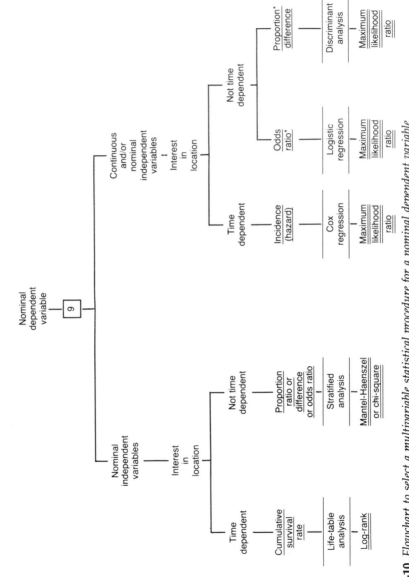

FIGURE 30-10 *Flowchart to select a multivariable statistical procedure for a nominal dependent variable (* = see Chap. 29 for discussion of methods for choosing between the point estimates).*

Glossary

ABSOLUTE RISK   The probability of an event occurring during a specified period of time. The absolute risk equals the relative risk times the average probability of the event during the same period of time if the risk factor is absent.

ACCURACY   The ability of a test to produce results that are close to the true measure of the phenomenon; lack of random or systematic error; precise and unbiased.

ADJUSTMENT   Techniques used after the collection of data to take into account or control for the effect of known or potential confounding variables (syn: control for, take into account, standardize).

ANALYSIS   The comparison of the outcome of the study and control groups.

ARTIFACTUAL DIFFERENCES OR CHANGES   Differences or changes in measures of occurrence that result from the way the disease or condition is measured, sought, or defined.

ASSESSMENT   The determination of the outcome of the study and control groups.

ASSIGNMENT   The selection of individuals for study and control groups.

ASSOCIATION   A relationship among two or more characteristics or other measurements beyond what would be expected by chance alone. When used to establish criterion No. 1 of contributory cause association implies that the two characteristics occur in the same individual more often than expected by chance alone.

ATTRIBUTABLE RISK PERCENTAGE   The percentage of the risk *among those with the risk factor* that is associated with the risk factor. If a cause and effect relationship exists, attributable risk is the percentage of a disease that can be expected to be eliminated among those with the risk factor, if the effect of the risk factor can be completely eliminated. (syn: attributable risk, attributable risk [exposed], etiological fraction [exposed], percentage risk reduction, protective efficacy rate).

BIAS   A condition that causes a result to depart from the true values in a consistent direction. The use of this term is limited to the result of defects in study design.

BLIND ASSESSMENT   The evaluation of the outcome for individuals without the person who makes the evaluation knowing whether the individuals were in the study group or the control group.

BLIND ASSIGNMENT   Occurs when individuals are assigned to a study group and a control group without the investigator or the subjects being aware of the group to which they are assigned. When both investigator and subjects are "blinded," the study is sometimes referred to as a *double-blind study*.

CASE-CONTROL   A study that begins by identifying individuals with a disease (cases) and individuals without a disease (controls). The cases and controls are identified without knowledge of an individual's exposure or nonexposure to factors being investigated. These factors are determined from existing information (syn: retrospective).

CASE FATALITY   The number of deaths due to a particular disease divided by the number of individuals diagnosed with the disease at the beginning of the time interval. The case fatality estimates the probability of eventually dying from the disease. A case fatality rate includes, in addition, the number of person-years as a unit of time in the denominator.

CHUNK SAMPLE   A subset from a population that is assembled because of the ease of collecting the data without regard for the degree to which the sample is random or representative of the population of interest.

COEFFICIENT OF DETERMINATION (R^2) The square of a correlation coefficient. This statistic indicates the proportion of the variation in one variable (the dependent variable) that is explained by knowing a value of one or more other variables (the independent variables).

COHORT   A group of individuals who share a common exposure, experience, or characteristic (see cohort study, cohort effect).

COHORT EFFECT   A change in rates that can be explained by the common experience or characteristic of a group or cohort of individuals. A cohort effect implies that current rates should not be directly extrapolated into the future.

COHORT STUDY   A study that begins by identifying individuals with and without a factor being investigated. These factors are identified without knowledge of which individuals have or will develop disease. Cohort studies may be concurrent or nonconcurrent (syn: prospective).

CONCURRENT COHORT STUDY   A cohort study in which an individual's group assignment is determined at the time that the study begins and the study and control group participants are followed forward in time to determine if the disease occurs (syn: prospective cohort study).

CONFIDENCE INTERVAL (95%)   In statistical terms, the range of numerical values within which we can be 95% confident the population value we are estimating lies (syn: interval estimate).

CONFOUNDING VARIABLE   A characteristic or variable that is distributed differently in the study and control groups and that affects the outcome being assessed. A confounding variable may be due to chance or bias. When it is due to bias in the assignment process, the resulting error is also called a *selection bias* (syn: confounder).

CONTINUOUS DATA   A type of data with an unlimited number of equally spaced values (e.g., diastolic blood pressure, cholesterol).

CONTRIBUTORY CAUSE   Contributory cause is established when all three of the following have been established: (1) the existence of an association between the cause and the effect, (2) the cause precedes the effect in time, and (3) altering the cause alters the probability of occurrence of the effect.

CONTROL GROUP   A group of persons used for comparison with a study group. Ideally, the control group is identical to the study group except that it does not possess the characteristic or has not been exposed to the treatment under study (syn: reference group).

CONTROLLED CLINICAL TRIAL   An investigation in which the investigator assigns individuals to study and control groups using a process known as *randomization* (syn: randomized clinical trial, experimental study).

CORRELATION   A statistic used for studying the strength of an association between two variables, each of which has been sampled using a representative or naturalistic method from a population of interest.

CROSS-SECTIONAL STUDY   A study that identifies individuals with and without the condition or disease under study and the characteristic or exposure of interest at the same point in time.

DEGREES OF FREEDOM   A parameter of many standard statistical distributions. Degrees of freedom allow us to take into account the number of population parameters that must be estimated from a sample in order to perform certain statistical procedures.

DEPENDENT VARIABLE   Generally, the outcome variable of interest in any type of research study. The outcome that one intends to explain or estimate.

DIRECT CAUSE   A contributory cause that is the most directly known cause of a disease (e.g., hepatitis B virus is a direct cause of hepatitis B infection, and unclean needles are an indirect cause). The direct cause is dependent on the current state of knowledge and may change as more immediate mechanisms are discovered.

DISTRIBUTION   Frequencies or relative frequencies of all possible values of a characteristic. Population and sample distributions can be described graphically or mathematically. One of the purposes of statistics is to estimate parameters of population distributions.

DOSE-RESPONSE RELATIONSHIP   A dose-response relationship is present if changes in levels of an exposure are associated with changes in the frequency of the outcome in a consistent direction. A dose-response relationship is a supportive criterion for contributory cause.

ECOLOGICAL FALLACY   The type of error that can occur when the existence of a group association is used to imply the existence of a relationship that does not exist at the individual level.

EFFECT   An outcome that is brought about, at least in part, by an etiological factor known as the cause.

EFFECT OF OBSERVATION   A type of bias that results when the process of observation alters the outcome of the study.

EFFECTIVENESS   The extent to which a treatment produces a beneficial effect when implemented under the usual conditions of clinical care for a particular group of patients.

EFFICACY   The extent to which a treatment produces a beneficial effect when assessed under the ideal conditions of an investigation. Efficacy is to therapy as contributory cause is to etiology of disease.

ESTIMATE   A value or range of values calculated from sample observations that are used to approximate a corresponding population value or parameter (also see interval estimate, point estimate).

EXTRAPOLATION   Conclusions drawn about the meaning of the study for a target population that includes types of individuals or data not represented in the study sample.

FALSE-NEGATIVE   An individual whose result on a test is negative but who has the disease or condition as determined by the gold standard.

FALSE-POSITIVE   An individual whose result on a test is positive but who does not have the disease or condition as determined by the gold standard.

GAUSSIAN DISTRIBUTION   A distribution of data assumed in many statistical procedures. The Gaussian distribution is a symmetrical, continuous, bell-shaped curve with its mean value corresponding to the highest point on the curve (syn: normal distribution).

GOLD STANDARD   The criterion used to unequivocally define the presence of a condition or disease under study.

GROUP ASSOCIATION   The situation in which a characteristic and a disease both occur more frequently in one group of individuals compared to another group of individuals. Group association does not necessarily imply that individuals with the characteristic are the same ones who have the disease (syn: ecological association, ecological correlation).

GROUP MATCHING   A matching procedure used during assignment in an investigation that selects study and control individuals in such a way that the groups have a nearly equal distribution of a particular variable or variables (syn: frequency matching).

INCIDENCE RATE   The rate at which new cases of disease occur per unit of time. The incidence rate is theoretically calculated as the number of individuals who develop the disease over a period of time divided by the total person-years at risk.

INDEPENDENT VARIABLE   Variables being measured to determine the corresponding measurement of the dependent variable in any type of research study. Independent variables define the conditions under which the dependent variable is to be examined.

INDIRECT CAUSE   A contributory cause that acts through a biological mechanism that is more closely related to the disease than it is to the direct cause. (e.g., unclean needles are an indirect contribution cause of hepatitis B; the hepatitis B virus is a direct contributory cause) (see direct cause).

INFERENCE   In statistical terminology, inference is the logical process that occurs during statistical significance testing (see statistical significance test).

INSTRUMENT ERROR   A bias in assessment that results when the testing instrument is not appropriate to the conditions of the study or is not accurate enough in measuring the study outcome.

INTEROBSERVER VARIATION   Variation in measurement by different individuals.

INTERPRETATION   The drawing of conclusions about the meaning of any differences found between the study group and the control group for those included in the investigation.

INTERVAL ESTIMATE   See confidence interval.

INTRAOBSERVER VARIATION   Variation in measurements by the same person at different times.

LEAD-TIME BIAS   An artifactual difference in rates that occurs when screening produces earlier diagnosis that does not lead to improved prognosis.

LIFE-TABLE METHOD   A method for organizing data that allows examination of the experience of one or more groups of individuals over time when some individuals are followed for longer periods of time than others (syn: Kaplan-Meier, Cutler-Ederer life-tables, cohort or clinical life-table). Distinct from cross-sectional or current life-tables that produce life-expectancy measurements.

MATCHING   The analysis together of two or more observations from the same individual or similar individuals. Pairing is a special type of matching where two observations are analyzed together.

MEAN   Sum of the measurements divided by the number of measurements being added together. The "center of gravity" of a distribution of observations. A special type of average.

MEDIAN   The mid-point of a distribution. The median is chosen so that half the data values occur above and half occur below the median.

MORTALITY RATE   A measure of the incidence of death. This rate is calculated as the number of deaths over a period of time divided by the number of individuals times the period of follow-up.

NATURAL EXPERIMENT   An investigation in which a change in a risk factor occurs in one group of individuals but not in a control group. As opposed to controlled clinical trials, in a natural experiment the change is not brought about by the intervention of an investigator.

NATURALISTIC SAMPLE   A set of observations obtained from a population in such a way that the sample distribution of independent variable values is representative of their distribution in the population.

NECESSARY CAUSE   A characteristic is a necessary cause if its presence is required to bring about or cause the disease.

NOMINAL DATA   A type of data with named categories. If nominal data has more than two categories they cannot be ordered (e.g. race, eye color). Nominal data requires more than one nominal variable if there are more than two potential categories.

NONCURRENT COHORT STUDY   A cohort study in which an individual's group assignment is determined by information existing at the time a study begins. The extreme of a nonconcurrent cohort study is one in which the outcome is subsequently determined from existing records (syn: retrospective cohort study).

NONPARAMETRIC STATISTICS   Statistical procedures that do not make assumptions about the distribution of parameters in the population being sampled. Nonparametric statistical methods are not free of assumptions such as the assumption of random sampling. They are most often used for ordinal data but may be used for continuous data converted to an ordinal scale.

NORMAL DISTRIBUTION   See Gaussian distribution.

NULL HYPOTHESIS   The assertion that no true association or difference between variables exists in the larger population from which the study samples are obtained.

NUMBER NEEDED TO TREAT   The reciprocal of the difference in risk. The number of patients, similar to the study patients who need to be treated to obtain one fewer bad outcome or one more good outcome.

ODDS RATIO   A measure of the degree or strength of an association applicable to all types of studies employing nominal data but usually applied to case-control and cross-sectional studies. The odds ratio for case-control and cross-sectional studies is measured as the odds of having the risk factor if the condition is present divided by the odds of having the risk factor if the condition is not present.

ONE-TAILED TEST   A statistical significance test in which deviations from the null hypothesis in only one direction are considered. Use of a one-tailed test implies that the investigator does not consider a true deviation in the opposite direction to be possible.

ORDINAL DATA   A type of data with a limited number of categories with an inherent ordering of the categories from lowest to highest. Ordinal data, however, say nothing about the spacing between categories (e.g., stage 1, 2, 3, 4 cancer).

OUTCOME   The end point of an investigation of the measurement being used in the assessment process. In case-control studies, outcome is a prior characteristic; in cohort studies and controlled clinical trials, the outcome or end point is a future event.

P VALUE   The probability of making an observation at least as extreme from the condition described in the null hypothesis as we observe in our data set if the null hypothesis were true. The P value is considered the "bottom line" in statistical significance testing.

PAIRING   A special form of matching in which each study individual is coupled or paired with a control group individual and their outcomes are compared. When pairing is used, special statistical methods should be used. These methods may increase the statistical power of the study.

PARAMETER   A value that summarizes the distribution of a large population. One of the purposes of statistical analysis is to estimate population parameters from sample observations.

POINT ESTIMATE   A single value calculated from sample observations that is used as the estimate of the population value, or parameter.

POPULATION   A large group often but not necessarily of individuals. In statistics, one attempts to draw conclusions about a population or populations by obtaining subsets or samples made up of individuals from the larger population(s).

POPULATION ATTRIBUTABLE RISK PERCENTAGE   The percentage of the risk among a community, *including individuals with and without a risk factor,* that is associated with exposure to a risk factor. Population attributable risk does not necessarily imply a cause and effect relationship (syn: attributable fraction [population], attributable proportion [population], etiological fraction [population]).

POWER   The ability of an investigation to demonstrate statistical significance when a true association or difference of a specified strength exists in the population being sampled (syn: statistical power, resolving power).

PRECISE   The lack of random or chance error (an imprecise measure can deviate from the true numerical value in either direction).

PREDICTIVE VALUE OF A NEGATIVE TEST   The proportion of those with a negative test who do not have the condition or disease as measured by the gold standard. This measure incorporates the prevalence of the condition or disease. Clinically, the predictive value of a negative test is the probability that an individual does not have the disease if the test is negative (syn: posttest probability).

PREDICTIVE VALUE OF A POSITIVE TEST   The proportion of those with a positive test who actually have the condition or disease as measured by the gold standard. This measure incorporates the prevalence of the condition or disease. Clinically, the predictive value of a positive test is the probability that an individual has the disease if the test is positive (syn: posttest probability).

PREVALENCE   The proportion of persons with a particular disease or condition at a point in time. Prevalence can also be interpreted as the probability that an individual selected at random from the population will be someone who has the disease or condition (syn: pretest probability).

PROBABILITY   A proportion in which the numerator contains the number of times an event occurs, and the denominator includes the number of times an event occurs plus the number of times it does not occur.

PROPORTION   A fraction in which the numerator contains a subset of the individuals contained in the denominator.

PROPORTIONATE MORTALITY RATIO   A fraction in which the numerator contains the number of individuals who die of a particular disease over a period of time, and the denominator contains the number of individuals dying from all diseases over the same period time.

PROSPECTIVE STUDY   See cohort study.

PURPOSIVE SAMPLE   A set of observations obtained from a population in such a way that the sample distribution of independent variable values is determined by the researcher and not necessarily representative of their distribution in the population.

RANDOMIZATION   A method of assignment in which individuals have a known, but not necessarily equal, probability of being assigned to a particular study or control group. As distinguished from random selection, the individuals being randomized may or may not be representative of a large population (syn: random assignment).

RANDOMIZED CLINICAL TRIAL   See controlled clinical trial.

RANDOM SELECTION   A method of obtaining a sample that ensures that each individual in the larger population has a known, but not necessarily equal, probability of being selected for the sample.

RANGE   The difference between the highest and lowest data values in a population or sample.

RANGE OF NORMAL   A measure of the range of values on a test among those without disease. Often the central 95% or the mean value for those without disease plus or minus two standard deviations.

RATE   Commonly used to indicate any measure of disease or outcome occurrence. From a statistical point of view, rates are those measures of disease occurrence that include time in the denominator (e.g., incidence).

RATIO   A fraction in which the numerator is not necessarily a subset of the denominator as opposed to a proportion.

RECALL BIAS   An assessment bias that occurs when individuals in one group are more likely to remember past effects than individuals in another of the study or control groups. Recall bias is especially likely when a case-control study involves serious disease and the characteristics under study are commonly occurring, subjectively remembered events.

REFERENCE GROUP   The group of presumably disease-free individuals from which a sample of individuals is acquired whose measurements on a test are used to establish a range of normal (syn: reference population).

REGRESSION TECHNIQUES   A series of statistical methods useful for describing the association between one dependent variable and one or more independent variables. Regression techniques are often used to perform adjustment for confounding variables.

REGRESSION TO THE MEAN   A statistical principle based on the fact that unusual events are unlikely to recur. By chance alone, measurements subsequent to an unusual measurement are likely to be closer to the mean. In addition there may be social or psychological factors that help force subsequent events back toward the mean.

RELATIVE RISK   A ratio of the probability of developing the outcome in a specified period of time if the risk factor is present divided by the probability of developing the outcome in that same period of time if the risk factor is not present. The relative risk is a measure of the strength or degree of association applicable to cohort and randomized clinical trials. In case-control studies, the odds ratio often can be used to approximate the relative risk.

REPORTING BIAS   An assessment bias that occurs when individuals in one group are more likely to report past events than individuals in another of the study or control groups. Reporting bias is especially likely to occur when one group is under disproportionate pressure to report confidential information.

REPRODUCIBILITY   The ability of a test to produce consistent results when repeated under the same conditions and interpreted without knowledge of the first test results (syn: reliability, repeatability).

RETROSPECTIVE STUDY   See case-control.

RISK   The probability of an event occurring during a specified period of time. The numerator of risk contains the number of individuals who develop the disease during the time period; the denominator contains the number of disease-free persons at the beginning of the time period.

RISK FACTOR   A characteristic or factor that has been shown to be associated with an increased probability of developing a condition or disease. A risk factor does not necessarily imply a cause and effect relationship. In this book, a risk factor will imply that at least an association has been established on an individual level.

ROBUST   A statistical procedure is robust if its assumptions can be violated without substantial effects on its conclusions.

SAMPLE   A subset of a larger population obtained for investigation to draw conclusions or make estimates about the larger population.

SAMPLING ERROR   An error introduced by chance differences between the estimate obtained in a sample and the true value in the larger population from which the sample was drawn. Sampling error is inherent in the use of sampling methods and is measured by the standard error.

SELECTION BIAS   A bias in assignment that occurs when the study and control groups are chosen so that they differ from each other by one or more factors that affect the outcome of the study. A special type of confounding variable that results from study design rather than chance (see confounding variable).

SENSITIVITY   The proportion of those with the disease or condition as measured by the gold standard who are positive by the test being studied (syn: positive in disease).

SPECIFICITY   The proportion of those without the disease or condition as measured by the gold standard who are negative by the test being studied (syn: negative in disease).

STANDARD DEVIATION   A commonly used measure of the spread or dispersion of data. The standard deviation squared is known as the variance.

STANDARD ERROR   The spread or dispersion of point estimates obtained from samples of a specified size.

STANDARDIZATION (OF A RATE)   An effort to take into account or adjust for the effects of a factor such as age or sex on the obtained rates (see adjustment).

STANDARDIZED MORTALITY RATIO   A fraction in which the numerator contains the observed number of deaths, and the denominator contains the number of deaths that would be expected based on a comparison population. A standard mortality ratio implies that indirect standardization has been used to control for confounders. Note that the terms *standardized mortality ratio* and *proportionate mortality ratio* are not synonymous.

STATISTIC   A value calculated from sample data that is used to estimate a value or parameter in the larger population from which the sample was obtained.

STATISTICAL SIGNIFICANCE TEST   A statistical technique for determining the probability that the association observed in a sample might occur by chance if there is no such difference or association in the larger parent population (syn: inference, hypothesis testing).

STRATIFICATION   In general, stratification means to divide into groups. Stratification might be used to refer to a process to control for differences in confounding variables by making separate estimates for groups of individuals who have the same values for the confounding variable. Stratification might also refer to a purposive sampling method that is designed to oversample rare categories of an independent variable.

STUDY GROUP   In a cohort or controlled clinical trial, a group of individuals who possess the characteristics or are exposed to the factors under study. In case-control or cross-sectional study, a group of individuals who have developed the disease or condition being investigated.

STUDY HYPOTHESIS   An assertion that an association exists between two or more variables in the population sampled. A study hypothesis can be one-tailed, considering associations in one direction only, or two-tailed, not specifying the direction of the association.

SUFFICIENT CAUSE   A characteristic is a sufficient cause if its presence in and of itself will bring about or cause the disease.

SUPPORTIVE CRITERIA   When contributory cause cannot be established, additional criteria can be used to develop a judgment regarding the existence of a contributory cause. These include strength of association, dose-response relationship, consistency of the relationship, and biologic plausibility (syn: adjunct, ancillary criteria).

TARGET POPULATION   The group of individuals to whom one wishes to apply or extrapolate the results of an investigation. The target population may be, and often is, different from the population from which the sample in an investigation is drawn.

TRUE-NEGATIVE   An individual who does not have the disease or condition as measured by the gold standard and has a negative test result.

TRUE-POSITIVE   An individual who has the disease or condition as measured by the gold standard and has a positive test result.

TWO-TAILED TEST   A statistical significance test in which deviations from the null hypothesis in either direction are considered. Use of a two-tailed test implies that the investigator was willing to consider deviations in either direction before data were collected.

TYPE I ERROR   An error that occurs when data demonstrate a statistically significant result when no true association or difference exists in the population. The alpha level is the size of the Type I error which will be tolerated—usually 5%.

TYPE II ERROR   An error that occurs when sample observations fail to demonstrate statistical significance when a true association or difference actually exists in the larger population(s).

UNBIASED   Lack of systematic error.

VALID   A measurement is valid if it is appropriate for the question being addressed; measures what it intends to measure.

VARIABLE   In its general usage variable refers to a characteristic for which measurements are made in a study. In strict statistical terminology a variable is the representative of those measurements in an analysis. Continuous or ordinal scale data is expressed using one variable as is nominal data with only two categories. However, nominal data with more than two categories must be expressed using more than one variable.

VARIANCE   See standard deviation.

Index

Absolute risk, defined, 56
Accuracy of diagnostic tests. *See* Diagnostic tests, accuracy of
Accuracy of sampling. *See* Samples/ sampling, accuracy of
Adjustment
  of data. *See* Data, adjustment of
  of range of normal in tests, 139-140, 145-146, 168
    false negatives/false positives and, 139-140
Aims of study, adequate definition of, 65, 73, 75
Analysis, 25-45
  according to the intention to treat, 102
  ACOVA. *See* Analysis, of covariance
  ANOVA. *See* Analysis, of variance
  bivariable, 263-287
  case control studies, 9, 10, 82-83
  cohort studies, 11, 12, 85
  of confidence intervals, 44-45
  confounding variables and, 25-26, 74, 76
  correlation, 275-277
  of covariance, 299-302, 313
  defined, 7, 8
  discriminant, 310, 314
  evaluation of, 74
  flaw-catching exercises, 82-83, 85, 89-90
  life table, 104-109, 307-308, 314
  multivariable, 289-314
  prior matching of individual and control groups and, 26-28
  probit, 311
  questions on, 76

  of randomized clinical trials, 11, 13, 103-107, 119-120, 123
  regression. *See* Regression methods (analysis)
  statistical significance testing, 28-45, 74, 76. *See also* Statistical significance test(s)
  stratified, 306, 308, 312
  univariable, 245-261
  of variance, 291-293, 295, 296, 298, 300, 302-304, 313-314
Artifactual changes/differences in rates. *See* Rate(s), artifactual changes in
Assessment of outcome, 19-24
  accurate, 21-22, 29
  appropriate measures of, 19-20, 74, 76
    criteria for, 20
  blind, 22-23
  case control studies, 9, 10, 19
  cohort studies, 11, 12, 19, 85, 89
  completeness of, 23-24
  criteria for valid measures of, 19-24
  defined, 7, 8
  flaw-catching exercises, 81-82, 89
  imprecise measurement/instrument error, 20-22
  incomplete follow-up, 23-24
  investigator bias/misinterpretation, 22-23
  observational process and, 20, 24, 73, 76
  questions on, 76
  randomized clinical trials, 11, 13
  recall bias, 21
  reporting bias, 21-22
  reports by individuals and, 21-22